T0259308

Infectious Diseases and Asthma

Guest Editors

SHYAM MOHAPATRA, PhD
GARY HELLERMANN, PhD

IMMUNOLOGY AND ALLERGY CLINICS OF NORTH AMERICA

www.immunology.theclinics.com

Consulting Editor
RAFEUL ALAM, MD, PhD

November 2010 • Volume 30 • Number 4

SAUNDERS an imprint of ELSEVIER, Inc.

W.B. SAUNDERS COMPANY
A Division of Elsevier Inc.

1600 John F. Kennedy Blvd., ● Suite 1800 ● Philadelphia, PA 19103-2899.

http://www.theclinics.com

IMMUNOLOGY AND ALLERGY CLINICS OF NORTH AMERICA Volume 30, Number 4
November 2010 ISSN 0889–8561, ISBN-13: 978-1-4377-2459-2

Editor: Patrick Manley

Immunology and Allergy Clinics of North America (ISSN 0889–8561) is published quarterly by Elsevier Inc., 360 Park Avenue South, New York, NY 10010-1710. Months of issue are February, May, August, and November. Periodicals postage paid at New York, NY and additional mailing offices. Subscription prices are $272.00 per year for US individuals, $392.00 per year for US institutions, $129.00 per year for US students and residents, $334.00 per year for Canadian individuals, $187.00 per year for Canadian students, $486.00 per year for Canadian institutions, $379.00 per year for international individuals, $486.00 per year for international institutions, $187.00 per year for international students. To receive student/resident rate, orders must be accompanied by name of affiliated institution, date of term, and the *signature* of program/residency coordinator on institution letterhead. Orders will be billed at individual rate until proof of status is received. Foreign air speed delivery is included in all *Clinics* subscription prices. All prices are subject to change without notice. **POSTMASTER**: Send address changes to *Immunology and Allergy Clinics of North America*, Elsevier Health Sciences Division, Subscription Customer Service, 3251 Riverport Lane, Maryland Heights, MO 63043. **Customer Service: 1-800-654-2452 (U.S. and Canada); 314-447-8871 (outside U.S. and Canada). Fax: 314-447-8029. E-mail: journalscustomerservice-usa@elsevier.com (for print support); journalsonlinesupport-usa@elsevier.com (for online support).**

Reprints. For copies of 100 or more, of articles in this publication, please contact the Commercial Reprints Department, Elsevier Inc., 360 Park Avenue South, New York, New York 10010-1710. Tel. (212) 633-3812, Fax: (212) 462-1935, e-mail: reprints@elsevier.com.

Immunology and Allergy Clinics of North America is covered in MEDLINE/PubMed (Index Medicus), Current Contents/Life Sciences, Science Citation Index, ISI/BIOMED, Chemical Abstracts, and EMBASE/Excerpta Medica.

Printed and bound by CPI Group (UK) Ltd, Croydon, CR0 4YY

Transferred to Digital Print 2011

Contributors

CONSULTING EDITOR

RAFEUL ALAM, MD, PhD
Veda and Chauncey Ritter Chair in Immunology, Professor, and Director, Division
of Immunology and Allergy, National Jewish Health; and University of Colorado
Health Sciences Center, Denver, Colorado

GUEST EDITORS

SHYAM MOHAPATRA, PhD, FAAAI
Mabel and Ellsworth Simmons Professor of Allergy and Immunology, Divisions of Allergy
and Immunology and Translational Medicine, Department of Internal Medicine, University
of South Florida College of Medicine; James A. Haley Veterans' Administration Hospital
Medical Center, Tampa, Florida

GARY HELLERMANN, PhD
Senior Biological Scientist, Divisions of Allergy and Immunology and Translational
Medicine, Department of Internal Medicine, University of South Florida College of
Medicine, Tampa, Florida

AUTHORS

PEDRO C. AVILA, MD
Associate Professor of Medicine, Division of Allergy-Immunology, Feinberg School
of Medicine, Northwestern University, Chicago, Illinois

SILVIO FAVORETO Jr, PhD, DDS
Research Associate Professor of Medicine, Biology Division, Cuesta College,
San Luis Obispo, California

JAMES E. GERN, MD
Departments of Pediatrics and Medicine, University of Wisconsin-Madison School
of Medicine and Public Health, Madison, Wisconsin

ALYSSA GREIMAN, BSc
Research Assistant, Division of Allergy-Immunology, Feinberg School of Medicine,
Northwestern University, Chicago, Illinois

GARY HELLERMANN, PhD
Senior Biological Scientist, Divisions of Allergy and Immunology and Translational
Medicine, Department of Internal Medicine, University of South Florida College of
Medicine, Tampa, Florida

DANIEL J. JACKSON, MD
Assistant Professor of Pediatrics, Department of Pediatrics, University of Wisconsin
School of Medicine and Public Health, Madison, Wisconsin

KIRSTEN M. KLOEPFER, MD
Departments of Pediatrics and Medicine, University of Wisconsin-Madison School of Medicine and Public Health, Madison, Wisconsin

MATTI KORPPI, MD, PhD
Professor, Pediatric Research Center, Tampere University and University Hospital, Tampere, Finland

MONICA KRAFT, MD
Professor of Medicine, Department of Medicine, Division of Pulmonary, Allergy and Critical Care Medicine, Duke University Medical Center, Durham, North Carolina

ROBERT F. LEMANSKE Jr, MD
Professor of Pediatrics and Medicine, Departments of Pediatrics and Medicine, University of Wisconsin School of Medicine and Public Health, Madison, Wisconsin

PETER MCERLEAN, PhD
Post-Doctoral Research Fellow, Division of Allergy-Immunology, Feinberg School of Medicine, Northwestern University, Chicago, Illinois

GREGORY METZ, MD
Medical Instructor, Department of Medicine, Division of Pulmonary, Allergy and Critical Care Medicine, Duke University Medical Center, Durham, North Carolina

E. KATHRYN MILLER, MD, MPH
Assistant Professor, Pediatric, Pulmonary, Allergy and Immunology, Department of Medicine, Vanderbilt University Medical Center, Vanderbilt Children's Hospital, Nashville, Tennessee

SHYAM MOHAPATRA, PhD, FAAAI
Mabel and Ellsworth Simmons Professor of Allergy and Immunology, Divisions of Allergy and Immunology and Translational Medicine, Department of Internal Medicine, University of South Florida College of Medicine; James A. Haley Veterans' Administration Hospital Medical Center, Tampa, Florida

R. STOKES PEEBLES Jr, MD
Associate Professor of Medicine, Division of Allergy, Pulmonary, and Critical Care Medicine, Department of Medicine, Vanderbilt University School of Medicine, Vanderbilt University Medical Center, Nashville, Tennessee

LOUIS A. ROSENTHAL, PhD
Scientist, Division of Allergy, Pulmonary and Critical Care Medicine, Department of Medicine, University of Wisconsin School of Medicine and Public Health, Madison, Wisconsin

BLAIR D. WESTERLY, MD
Resident in Internal Medicine, Department of Medicine, Vanderbilt University School of Medicine, Vanderbilt University Medical Center, Nashville, Tennessee

TERIANNE WONG, BSc
Department of Molecular Medicine, University of South Florida College of Medicine, Tampa, Florida

Contents

There has been significant progress in our knowledge about the relationship between infectious disease and the immune system in relation to asthma, but many unanswered questions still remain. Respiratory tract infections such as those caused by respiratory syncytial virus and rhinovirus during the first 2 years of life are still clearly associated with later wheezing and asthma, but the mechanism has not been completely worked out. Is there an "infectious march" triggered by infection in infancy that progresses to disease pathology or are infants who contract respiratory infections predisposed to developing asthma? This review focuses on the common themes in the interaction between microbes and the immune system, and presents a critical appraisal of the evidence to date. The various mechanisms whereby microbes alter the immune response and how this might influence asthma are discussed along with new and promising clinical practices for prevention and therapy. Recent advances in using sensitive polymerase chain reaction detection methods have allowed more rigorous testing of the causality hypothesis of virus infection leading to asthma, but the evidence is still equivocal. Various exceptions and inconsistencies in the clinical trials are discussed in light of new guidelines for subject inclusion/exclusion in hopes of providing some standardization. Despite past failures in vaccination and disappointing results of some clinical trials, the new strategies for prophylaxis including RNA interference and targeted delivery of microbicides offer a large dose of hope to a world suffering from an increasing incidence of asthma as well as a huge burden of health care cost and loss of quality of life.

Asthma exacerbations are precipitated primarily by respiratory virus infection and frequently require immediate medical intervention. Studies of childhood and adult asthma have implicated a wide variety of respiratory viruses in exacerbations. By focusing on both RNA and DNA respiratory viruses and some newly identified viruses, this review illustrates the diversity and highlights some of the uncertainties that exist in our understanding of virus-related asthma exacerbations.

There is increasing evidence that experiencing viral wheezing illnesses early in life, especially in conjunction with allergic sensitization, is an important risk factor for the onset of asthma. In this review, the potential advantages and disadvantages of using rodent models of virus-induced chronic airway dysfunction to investigate the mechanisms by which early-life viral respiratory tract infections could initiate a process leading to chronic airway dysfunction and the asthmatic phenotype are discussed. The potential usefulness of rodent models for elucidating the viral, host, environmental, and developmental factors that might influence these processes is emphasized. There is a need for the continued development of rodent models of early-life viral respiratory tract infections that include the development of chronic airway dysfunction, the capacity to add components of allergic sensitization and allergic airway inflammation, and the ability to address both immunologic and physiologic consequences. Investigation of these rodent models should complement the research from pediatric cohort studies and begin to bring us closer to understanding the role of viral respiratory tract infections in the inception of childhood asthma.

Viral respiratory illnesses associated with wheezing are extremely common during early life and remain a frequent cause of morbidity and hospitalization in young children. Although many children who wheeze with respiratory viruses during infancy outgrow the problem, most children with asthma and reductions in lung function at school age begin wheezing during the first several years of life. Whether symptomatic viral infections of the lower respiratory tract are causal in asthma development or simply identify predisposed children remains a controversial issue. Wheezing illnesses caused by respiratory syncytial virus (RSV), particularly those severe enough to lead to hospitalization, have historically been associated with an increased risk of asthma at school age. However, with the development of molecular diagnostics, human rhinovirus (HRV) wheezing illnesses have been recognized more recently as a stronger predictor of school-age asthma than RSV. In this article, the authors review the impact of virus infections during early life, focusing primarily on RSV and HRV, and their potential roles in asthma inception.

Respiratory syncytial virus (RSV), a single-stranded RNA virus of the Paramyxoviridae family, is a major cause of bronchiolitis in infants and is also conjectured to be an early-life influence on the development of asthma. Although the data supporting a role for RSV in bronchiolitis in children are robust and evidence to support its role in juvenile asthmatics exists, RSV's role in asthma pathogenesis in adults is not as clearly defined. The authors review the literature to further elucidate RSV's impact on adult asthmatics, including its importance as a cause of asthma exacerbations.

They examine the morbidity associated with RSV infection and how the immune response may differ between adult asthmatics and nonasthmatics. They review the responses by specific cell types from adults with asthma that are stimulated by RSV. They also consider the role of early-life exposure to RSV and its contribution to asthma in adults. Lastly, they review the mechanisms by which RSV evades normal host immune responses and subverts these responses to its benefit.

Asthma is the most common chronic disease of childhood, affecting 10% to 15% of all children. Several different stimuli including allergens, tobacco smoke, certain drugs, and viral or bacterial infections are known to exacerbate asthma symptoms. Among these triggers, viruses are frequent inducers of asthma exacerbations, with human rhinoviruses being the most common in children and adults. This article describes the different species of this virus and their roles as major triggers of asthma exacerbations.

Clinical research findings indicate that there are synergistic interactions between allergy and viral infection that cause increased severity of asthma exacerbations. This article summarizes the current literature linking these 2 risk factors for asthma exacerbation, and reviews experimental data suggesting potential mechanisms for interactions between viral infection and allergy that cause asthma exacerbations. In addition, the authors discuss clinical evidence that treatment of allergic inflammation could help to reduce the frequency and severity of virus-induced exacerbations of asthma.

Streptococcus pneumoniae, *Haemophilus influenzae* and *Moraxella catarrhalis* seem to have no role in asthma in children. *Mycoplasma pneumoniae* and *Chlamydophila pneumoniae* can induce wheezing and cause asthma exacerbations in children, and chronic *Chlamydophila* infections may even participate in asthma pathogenesis. However, studies have failed to show any benefits from antibiotics for incipient or stable pediatric asthma, as well as for asthma exacerbations in children. Exposure to antibiotics in infancy has been an independent risk factor of later asthma in many studies. A recent study applying molecular biology methods to lower airway samples provided preliminary evidence that lower airways are not sterile but have their own protective microbiota, which can be disturbed in lung diseases like asthma.

Mycoplasma pneumoniae and *Chlamydophila pneumoniae* are atypical bacteria that are frequently found in patients with asthma. A definitive diagnosis of infection is often difficult to obtain because of limitations with sampling and detection. Numerous animal studies have outlined mechanisms by which these infections may promote allergic lung inflammation and airway remodeling. In addition, there is mounting evidence from human studies suggesting that atypical bacterial infections contribute to asthma exacerbations, chronic asthma, and disease severity. The role of antimicrobials directed against atypical bacteria in asthma is still under investigation.

RELATED INTEREST

Infectious Disease Clinics of North America (Volume 24, Issue 3, Pages 541–844 ,
September 2010)
Emerging Respiratory Infections in the 21st Century
Alimuddin Zumla, FRCP, PhD(Lond), FRCPath, Wing-Wai Yew, MBBS,
FRCP (Edinb), FCCP, David S.C. Hui, MD(UNSW), FRACP, FRCP, *Guest Editors*

THE CLINICS ARE NOW AVAILABLE ONLINE!

Access your subscription at:
www.theclinics.com

Foreword
Infection and Asthma

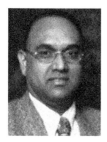

Rafeul Alam, MD, PhD
Consulting Editor

Infection has always been suspected to play a pivotal role in the pathogenesis and/or clinical course of asthma. Epidemiological studies have demonstrated an increased risk for atopy and asthma in children having recurrent infections or having infection with a specific microbe. Significant progress has been made in understanding the mechanism by which infection could augment an allergic immune response. The progress in the past was in part delayed by the dogma of Th1-Th2 antagonism. Allergic diseases represent a Th2 response, whereas infection typically elicits a Th1 response. Thus, it was conceptually difficult to reconcile a positive effect of infection on allergic inflammation. It should be stated that some publications had indicated a coexistence and even cooperation between Th1 and Th2 in asthma and atopic dermatitis. With the emergence of the concept of T-helper cell plasticity, it is now conceptually easier to imagine how infection could fuel an allergic response and transform the allergic phenotype into a complex one. For example a Th2 cell might transition into a phenotype that presents some features of Th2 and Th17 or even Th2 and Th1. The phenotype might resolve completely or partially after the infection. If the resolution is only partial, it would be now possible to identify the mixed phenotype and elucidate the contribution of this mixed phenotype to asthma.

With the progress in gene sequencing technology and microbiome analyses, it is likely that we will see more and more microbial species being recovered from the airways from asthmatic patients. The challenge is to distinguish the physiologic flora from the pathologic ones and then elucidate the immunologic consequences. This issue of *Immunology and Allergy Clinics* is devoted to the role of infection in asthma. Drs Mohapatra and Hellermann, two leaders in the field, have invited an outstanding group of scientists and

Supported by NIH grants RO1 AI059719 and AI68088, PPG HL 36577, and NO1 HHSN272200700048C.

0889-8561/10/$ – see front matter © 2010 Elsevier Inc. All rights reserved.
immunology.theclinics.com

clinicians. The result is a state-of-the-art presentation on various aspects of infection in asthma.

Rafeul Alam, MD, PhD
Division of Allergy and Immunology
National Jewish Health and University of Colorado Denver Health Sciences Center
1400 Jackson Street
Denver, CO 80206, USA

E-mail address:
alamr@njc.org

Preface

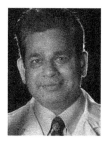 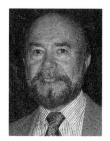

Shyam Mohapatra, PhD   Gary Hellermann, PhD
Guest Editors

Physicians and patients both have recognized a connection between asthma and respiratory infections since the disease was first described over two thousand years ago. The link has held throughout medical history until today; we recognize that about 80% of all asthma attacks can be associated with respiratory viral infections. We know a great deal more today than clinicians did in Hippocrates' time about the mechanism of asthma pathogenesis and pathology but the picture is still not complete. The sequencing of the human genome ushered in a decade of intense research into the genetics of disease and we have made great advances, but a complex illness like asthma whose etiology involves individual differences in immune responses, as well as an array of environmental factors from microbial infection to tobacco smoke, has proven an exceptionally tough nut to crack.

It all started with the discovery of respiratory syncytial virus (RSV)–specifically in the 1960s, when the connection between RSV infection and asthma became apparent. A depiction of the results from one of the earliest studies is illustrated in the accompanying figure (**Fig. 1**), which elegantly shows the connection between infection and asthma. Those individuals who suffered a bout of RSV bronchiolitis clearly had a greater chance of having later asthma attacks. Over the years other viruses such as rhinovirus and metapneumovirus have been implicated in asthma.

While asthma can be controlled in most cases through existing drugs, there is still a need for developing new therapies based on a person's individual phenotype and this requires delving into the cellular and molecular details behind the results we obtain from clinical trials. No one questions that there is a connection between the etiology of asthma and the occurrence of respiratory infections, but a clear picture of the mechanisms involved and the variations that can occur in different individuals have yet to be attained. It is hoped that this compendium of recent advances in the field of asthma pathology and respiratory infections will help to define the problems, provide the reader with the current state of research, and stimulate fruitful discussions and new hypotheses to fuel future discoveries.

In the introductory article, Wong, Hellermann, and Mohapatra provide an overview of the common themes in the interaction between microbes and the immune system.

Immunol Allergy Clin N Am 30 (2010) xiii–xviii
doi:10.1016/j.iac.2010.09.014   immunology.theclinics.com

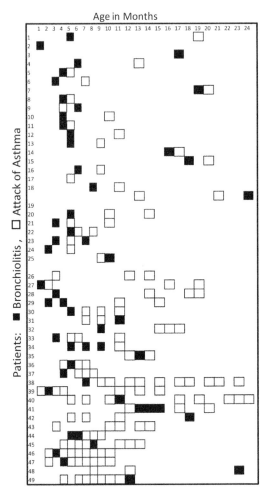

Fig. 1. Connection between RSV bronchiolitis and asthma attack. (*Adapted from* Hyde, JS, and Saed, AM. Acute bronchiolitis and the asthmatic child. J Asthma Res 1966;4:137–54; with permission.)

They present and evaluate the evidence for an "infectious march" beginning in infancy, describe the various possible mechanisms of microbial influence in asthma, and discuss new and promising clinical practices for prevention and therapy. Recent data obtained by utilizing sensitive PCR detection methods have allowed more rigorous clinical testing of the causality hypothesis of virus infection leading to asthma, but the evidence is still equivocal. Determining the "asthmagenic" potential of the many different types of bacteria and viruses that can colonize the respiratory tract is a daunting challenge. The important clinical trials are reviewed and various exceptions and inconsistencies in the results are discussed in light of new information on the inflammatory immune responses to microbial attack. The existing guidelines for subject inclusion/exclusion, types of outcome chosen, and data analysis are examined in hopes of providing some standardization. Despite past failures in vaccination and disappointing results of some clinical trials, the new strategies for prophylaxis including RNA interference, targeted microbicides, and inhibition of viral proteins offer a large dose of hope to a world suffering from an increasing incidence of asthma and a huge burden of health care cost and loss of quality of life.

The discussion continues with an article by Drs Kloepfer and Gern on the allergic asthmatic and their particular responses to viral respiratory infections. Allergen exposure is a common cause of asthma attacks, and when accompanied by a viral respiratory infection, the symptoms can be much more severe. The majority of asthma exacerbations have been found to also involve viral infections and much research has been done to define and understand the synergy between these two triggers of asthma exacerbation. An effective host antiviral response requires interferon production and expression of interferon response genes, and individual differences in the virus-neutralizing capability may occur under conditions of allergen exposure to increase the risk of an exacerbation and the severity of the attack. The combination of allergen sensitivity and exposure and virus infection, especially with rhinovirus, is frequently seen in children hospitalized for exacerbation. Recent studies using more sensitive detection methods have shown that rhinovirus can penetrate to the lower airways where it could interact with inflammation caused by allergen exposure. Underproduction of interferons or individual polarization toward a T helper cell 2-like cytokine environment could fuel the synergy seen in virus/allergen cases.

Dr Miller provides some highly interesting new information about the recently discovered species of human rhinovirus known as HRVC. More than 100 serotypes of the common cold virus have been identified over the years, but with the advent of more sensitive detection methods such as quantitative reverse-transcriptase PCR, the role of HRV in human diseases such as asthma has proven to be much greater than previously thought. Evidence is accumulating that shows HRV is more frequently associated with exacerbations than is RSV and that HRV may be linked to inception of asthma in children. HRVC is a genetically distinct species that is difficult to culture. Quantitative PCR methods, however, allow positive identification in sputum or nasal swabs. Some studies using these PCR methods have shown HVRC to be associated with a large proportion of hospitalizations for upper and lower respiratory illness, but other studies have shown no difference between HRVA, -B, and -C. As with nearly everything in asthma pathology, the answers are not simple or clear-cut and more work is definitely needed. Whether or not HRVC turns out to be more "asthmagenic" than other viruses remains to be determined.

Continuing with the theme of viral association in asthma inception, Drs Jackson and Lemanske explore the knotty question of whether viral bronchiolitis in infancy leads to asthma in childhood or if cellular and molecular conditions exist that predispose an individual to suffer both severe bronchiolitis and later asthma. Needless to say, the jury is still out on this matter, but are we closer to an unequivocal answer? The problem as usual lies in translating the in vitro and animal results to human trials. This article discusses in detail the clinical evidence related to the various hypotheses. All children are infected with respiratory viruses, but only some of the children who suffer viral bronchiolitis go on to develop wheezing and asthma that persist into adulthood. It may be informative to investigate the proteomics of those who "outgrow" their asthma with a view to teasing out the differences that preserve them from disease. More clinical studies of specific age groups, with long-term follow-up and tracking of molecular markers of inflammation and immunity, are needed to finally put this issue to rest.

Drs Westerly and Peebles survey the literature and offer up a cogent discussion about the role of RSV infection in the pathogenesis and progression of asthma in adults. The immune responses of asthmatics are different from those of nonasthmatics and we need to understand how this relates to respiratory virus susceptibility, severity of infection, and risk of exacerbation. One important consideration that needs to be addressed in RSV studies is that of seasonality, since unlike HRV, RSV has clear peaks of infection in the fall and winter. Here again, the authors emphasize the importance of using the sensitive and specific quantitative PCR method for virus detection. The elderly person is commonly at greater risk of pneumonia from respiratory virus infections than younger adults are and RSV is estimated to cause about 10,000 deaths per year in the over-65 age group. The immune system is not very good at curbing RSV infections and the reason for this seems to lie in RSV's ability to block the host cell's antiviral interferon defense system. Within hours after infecting a mucosal epithelial cell, the earliest RSV proteins, nonstructural protein-1 (NS1) and -2 (NS2), have been synthesized and are going to work to block expression of interferon and consequently the interferon-responsive genes. The viral proteins also prevent apoptosis of virally infected cells, allowing replication to proceed and titers to rise so that additional cells can be infected. The authors provide a detailed review of the changes and differences in cytokine levels, inflammatory mediators, and cellular profiles relating to RSV infection and exacerbation in asthmatics versus nonasthmatics.

The literature about the effects of a variety of less common respiratory viruses on asthma along with some newly identified virus candidates is reviewed and discussed by Dr McErlean, Ms Greiman, and Drs Favoreto and Avila. The viruses addressed include human metapneumovirus (HMPV; described pre-SARS), the human rhinovirus species C (HRVC), human coronaviruses (HCoVs) -NL63 and -HKU1, human bocavirus (HBoV), and the KI and WU polyoma-viruses (KIPyV and WUPyV). Some of the interesting questions reviewed by the authors include whether one virus such as HRV can suppress the replication of another such as influenzavirus, how asthma phenotype might affect colonization by specific viruses, and how differences in virus serotypes alter the risk of exacerbation or the severity of the reaction. The application of highly sensitive tests such as quantitative PCR for virus detection has demonstrated that coinfection with more than one virus is common, yet it is intriguing that this does not appear to increase the severity of an associated exacerbation. The enhanced detection capability has resulted in the detection of some newly identified viruses ("NIVs") among which were two types of polyoma virus discovered in 2007 associated with acute respiratory infections, bronchiolitis, and pneumonia. Whether these NIVs play any part in asthma pathogenesis or exacerbation has not yet been determined but they are especially interesting because there is evidence that they can exist in a latent form in cells and be reactivated under certain conditions.

Dr Rosenthal discusses the pros and cons of using mice and rats as models to study human asthma. The anatomy and physiology of the rodent respiratory system and their immune responses are different from those of humans. Other animal asthma models include guinea pigs, cotton rats, sheep, and nonhuman primates. The use of inbred rodent strains decreases the variability in results due to genotype. What constitutes an "ideal" rodent model? (1) The capability of studying the effects of infections and allergen sensitivity on asthma development, (2) the ability to test host genetic factors, (3) being able to look at the relationship between development of the immune system and pulmonary physiology, (4) the means to address changes in the airways due to chronic inflammation, and (5) changes due to immune senescence. The problems with limited replication of human viruses in rodents is partially solved by using rodent viruses such as mengovirus and sendai virus but these viruses may behave differently from their human counterparts. The use of gene-knockout strains of mice provides data about involvement of specific ligands, receptors, and enzymes in response to viral infection and development of asthma, and the use of conditional and inducible knockouts has further refined this method. Rodent models are also amenable to dose-response studies with environmental challenges such as tobacco smoke or diesel exhaust particles that would be unethical to do on humans. The short lifespan of the rodent makes it especially useful for aging and developmental studies.

The influence of specific bacterial infections on the pathogenesis of asthma is reviewed and evaluated by Dr Korppi. Bacteria such as *Mycoplasma pneumoniae* and *Chlamydophila pneumoniae* are associated with asthma exacerbations but antibiotics seem to be of little use in preventing them. Despite the hygiene hypothesis, the results confirm that early-life colonization with bacterial pathogens is not beneficial. However, the lower airways appear to have their own normal microbiota that is altered in asthmatics. Changes in the normal flora in childhood may affect asthma susceptibility. In fact, *C pneumoniae* may cause an occult chronic infection and inflammation in the airways and participate in the inception or pathogenesis of asthma. Increased sensitivity of detection methods may reveal infection where none was seen before. The new techniques have also shown us that the normal microbiota of humans is much more varied than earlier believed.

Drs Metz and Kraft expand upon the problems surrounding the effects of atypical infections with *M pneumoniae* and *C pneumoniae* on asthma susceptibility and exacerbation. There is emerging evidence to suggest that atypical bacterial infections are positively correlated with asthma exacerbations, chronic asthma, and severity of disease. Significant limitations exist in evaluating atypical bacterial infections in the lung due to difficulties with sampling and detection. The mechanisms of infection and the host responses as they relate to asthma inception and pathology are presented, followed by clinical evidence for involvement of atypical bacterial infection in exacerbations. The data support the idea that infection with atypical bacteria is associated with a worsening of asthma symptoms, especially during exacerbation, and with the development of chronic asthma. The bacterial attack on respiratory cells, cytokine involvement, oxidative stress, and epithelial cell denudation are all factors that are evaluated for their potential role in worsening asthma symptoms. Each bacterial type possesses unique mechanisms of action and the authors attempt to relate this to the observed effects on asthma. Antibiotics such as clarithromycin and roxithromycin have been tested with a view to reducing asthma exacerbations through reductions in bacterial colonization but results have been mixed.

In conclusion, the role of infection in asthma inception and pathogenesis has become clearer in the past decade but clinicians and basic scientists still have a way to go before all the details are worked out. The greatest hope for the future lies in the accessibility of a wonderful array of new tools from quantitative real-time PCR to 4D confocal microscopy and new types of microarrays. The tools are only as good as the minds that wield them, however, and it is hoped that this review of the asthma literature in relation to microbial attack will serve to stimulate thought that translates into action at the bench and new therapies in the clinic.

Shyam Mohapatra, PhD
Divisions of Allergy and Immunology and Translational Medicine
Department of Internal Medicine
University of South Florida College of Medicine
12908 USF Health Drive
Tampa, FL 33612, USA
James A. Haley Veterans' Administration Hospital Medical Center
13000 Bruce B. Downs Boulevard
Tampa, FL 33612, USA

Gary Hellermann, PhD
Divisions of Allergy and Immunology and Translational Medicine
Department of Internal Medicine
University of South Florida College of Medicine
12908 USF Health Drive
Tampa, FL 33612, USA

E-mail addresses:
smohapat@health.usf.edu (S. Mohapatra)
ghellerm@health.usf.edu (G. Hellermann)

The Infectious March: The Complex Interaction Between Microbes and the Immune System in Asthma

Terianne Wong, BSc[a], Gary Hellermann, PhD[b,c], Shyam Mohapatra, PhD[b,c,d],*

KEYWORDS

- Infection • Virus • Bacteria • Asthma • Inflammation
- Signaling • Mechanism

Like asthma itself, the association between respiratory infections and the inflammatory immune response is complex and incompletely understood. One can clearly see the effects of infections on wheezing, asthma inception, and exacerbations, but dissecting out the mechanistic details is the challenge confronting research in this decade. As always, it is hoped that a more complete understanding of the cells, cytokines, and signaling pathways involved, along with knowledge of the temporal progression of events and the role of regulatory factors such as microRNAs, will lead to more effective treatments, individualized to the patient.

Asthma afflicts more than 300 million individuals of all ages and ethnic groups, and results in approximately 250,000 deaths worldwide. More than 7 million children younger than 18 years have been diagnosed with asthma in the United States alone.[1] In 2003, asthma-related hospitalizations neared 500,000 in the United States and the annual direct medical expenses associated with asthma care were $12.7 to $15.6 billion.[2,3] According to a cross-sectional international study conducted from 2002 to

[a] Department of Molecular Medicine, University of South Florida College of Medicine, Bruce B. Downs Boulevard, Tampa, FL 33612, USA

[b] Division of Allergy and Immunology, Department of Internal Medicine, University of South Florida College of Medicine, 12908 USF Health Drive, Tampa, FL 33612, USA

[c] Division of Translational Medicine, Department of Internal Medicine, University of South Florida College of Medicine, 12908 USF Health Drive, Tampa, FL 33612, USA

[d] James A. Haley Veterans' Administration Hospital Medical Center, 13000 Bruce B. Downs Boulevard, Tampa, FL 33612, USA

* Corresponding author. Division of Allergy and Immunology, Department of Internal Medicine, University of South Florida College of Medicine, 12908 USF Health Drive, Tampa, FL 33612.

E-mail address: smohapat@health.usf.edu

Immunol Allergy Clin N Am 30 (2010) 453–480
doi:10.1016/j.iac.2010.09.008
0889-8561/10/$ – see front matter. Published by Elsevier Inc.

2003 by the International Study of Asthma and Allergies in Childhood (ISAAC), the prevalence of asthma symptoms reported in the 6- to 7-year-old age group increased significantly among 59% of the centers examined[4]; furthermore, the national surveillance report in 2007 identified a substantial increase in asthma attacks within the past 2 decades.[5]

In addition to the direct impact that asthma has on quality of life and health care costs among young populations, there is growing evidence for the existence of an asthmatic phenotype associated with increased susceptibility to respiratory tract infections (RIs) attributed to virus, particularly human rhinovirus (HRV) and respiratory syncytial virus (RSV).[6,7] Other respiratory viruses and certain atypical bacteria are also suspected of playing a part in airway inflammation and asthma pathogenesis.[8,9] In this article, the authors explore the mechanisms by which viral and bacterial infections trigger asthma exacerbations, look for similarities and differences, and discuss how some new therapeutic strategies are attempting to target these areas.

CORRELATIONS BETWEEN RESPIRATORY TRACT INFECTION AND WHEEZY BRONCHITIS AND ASTHMA

Advances in biotechnology in the 1990s have now provided diagnosticians with ultrasensitive methods such as quantitative real-time polymerase chain reaction (PCR) for identifying respiratory tract pathogens.[10,11] Nucleic acid sequence-based amplification (NASBA)[12] and high-throughput microarray chips, such as the Virochip,[13] have increased data collection by orders of magnitude. Early epidemiologic studies frequently suffered from variable viral isolation rates[14] and had to rely on tissue culture and serology for the detection of HRV, RSV, human influenza virus (IF), human parainfluenzavirus (HPIV), human metapneumovirus (HMPV), enterovirus, *Mycoplasma pneumoniae*, *Chlamydia pneumoniae*,[15] pneumococcal strains, and *Haemophilus influenzae*.[16,17] Microbial pathogens are usually more abundant in nasopharyngeal aspirates (NPA) from children and adults with active asthma.[17–19] Due to technological limitations and variable clinical criteria for diagnosing asthma,[14] observations from some early studies showed only weak correlations between respiratory infections and wheezy bronchitis and asthma.[20] Total viral isolation rates of RSV, HRV, and HPIV in children younger than 15 years were as low as 14.2% (38/267 children)[18] to as high as 45% (22/72 children)[17] during hospital admissions or reported asthma attacks. Despite the limitations, these early studies identified important factors that influence certain virus isolation rates, including patient readmission status and season of illness,[18] sensitivity of detection method,[14] environmental exposures such as parental smoking,[21] and patient age.[22] The controversial question of whether viral infections cause asthma exacerbations or if the asthma phenotype enhances susceptibility to infectious disease was still not answered.

One of the earliest longitudinal surveys, the Roehampton study conducted in the United Kingdom by Horn and colleagues,[23] spanned 1967 to 1972 and provided key information regarding potential changes in the types of pathogens isolated at different seasons and ages. Despite the lack of high-tech tools such as PCR and microarrays, the extensive study found that HRV, HPIV, and RSV were the predominant infectious agents in 614 isolates. RSV infection was highest among children younger than 4 years and occurred most often during winter months, whereas HRV illnesses occurred at all seasons and ages. Recent reports that use PCR and more sensitive methods generally confirm the findings of the Roehampton study.[7,24,25] The frequent detection of respiratory tract pathogens during acute lower respiratory bronchitis[26,27] suggests microbial pathogens trigger airway inflammation and stimulate leukocyte infiltration. More importantly, certain populations of children wheeze after a viral infection but show no symptoms of wheeze between viral infections, suggesting an immediate correlation between asthmatic phenotype and respiratory infections.[28] Although a multitude of factors, such as genetics, environment, weather, and atopic sensitization, could trigger asthma attacks, microbial pathogens have a potential for contributing to both persistent and episodic asthma attacks.

CAUSAL DIRECTION OF RESPIRATORY INFECTIONS IN ASTHMA: CLINICAL STUDIES IN CHILDREN

Birth cohort and longitudinal studies conducted in the last 2 decades also support the findings from Horn and colleagues.[23] In Perth, Australia, Kusel and colleagues[29] followed 236 infants from birth to their first year of life to assess the incidence of acute respiratory illnesses (ARIs) of viral or bacterial origin. Collecting NPA samples and using PCR for viral detection, the Perth study identified HRV, RSV, human coronavirus (HCoV), HPIV, and IF as the predominant respiratory pathogens associated with ARIs. In control children, who were healthy and asymptomatic, 24% of the NPA samples were positive for viral agent whereas viruses were present in 69% of the infected children. HRV was the most frequent virus identified with all 3 forms of ARI, including upper respiratory illness (URI), lower respiratory illness without wheeze (nwLRI), and lower respiratory illness with wheeze (wLRI). The attributable risk associated with wLRI, which is a measure of the degree to which a specific pathogen contributes to the severity of the respiratory illness, was highest for HRV and RSV, at 39% and 12%, respectively.[29] In a 5-year follow-up of the original Perth birth cohort, HRV- and RSV-associated wheeze with LRI were correlated with statistical significance to current or persistent wheeze, and current asthma later in life.[7] Skin prick tests helped categorize the remaining 198 children into the following groups: never atopic, atopic by age of 2 years, or atopic after 2 years. Combining ARI histories and status of atopic sensitization, children who were atopic by age 2 and had acquired wLRI HRV infections were found to have the greatest likelihood of developing wheeze by age 5 years. Odds ratios associated with this group nearly doubled when more than one wLRI was reported. The cohort studies by Merci and colleagues[7] provide evidence that HRV-induced wLRI and early sensitization are risk factors for current and persistent wheeze and asthma by the age of 5 years.

A report in 2008 by Jackson and colleagues[30] further supports a correlation between wheezy rhinovirus infections and the development of asthma in children younger than 6 years. Among 259 children examined in the study known as Childhood Origins of ASThma (COAST) in Madison, Wisconsin, 73 children developed childhood asthma by their sixth year. Wheezing illnesses attributed to either HRV or RSV in their third year of life increased their risk of developing asthma by age 6; in particular, 90% of children who had wheezy HRV-induced illness by age 3 subsequently became asthmatic by age 6 years. HRV-induced wheezing observed within the first, second, and third years of life increased the risk for asthma by the age of 6, and led to the conclusion that rhinovirus-associated illnesses during infancy are early predictors of subsequent development of asthma by age 6 years. In agreement with Merci and colleagues[7] and Stein and colleagues,[31] respiratory illnesses without wheeze were not statistically correlated with the development of asthma at age 6 years. Several longitudinal studies implicated HRV as a prominent viral pathogen in asthma etiology.

The causal direction of RSV-induced illness with asthma appears to be more difficult to define because the severity of RSV-induced disease appears to be affected by age,

Table 1
Clinical studies investigating respiratory tract infections in adults

Location	Study Period	Population Studied	Method for Detection	Pathogens Identified	Summary of Results
Wellington, New Zealand[22]	Prospective cohort; Jan 1984–Dec 1984	31 atopic asthmatic adults (15–56 y)	NPA for IF, cell culture, serology, electron microscopy	RSV, HRV, IF, HPIV, AdV, Herpes simplex, Enterovirus	60% of severe asthma exacerbations associated with viruses
Nottingham, UK[6]	Case-control; Sep 1993–Dec 1993	76 asthmatic adults (26–47 y) and cohabitating partners without asthma	NPA for PCR	HRV	Asthmatics with significantly longer and more frequent LRI
San Francisco, US[13,43]	Prospective cohort; Fall 2001–Dec 2004	53 adults with asthma, 30 without asthma	PCR, viral culture, and Virochip microarray	HRV, HCoV, RSV, HMPV, HPIV, IF	98% concordance with PCR and microarray; HRV most common with >20 serotypes

environment, and atopy. **Tables 1** and **2** summarize the study designs, population groups, and types of respiratory tract pathogens isolated in international clinical studies of adults and children from the 1970s to the current time. Four Swedish cohort studies conducted by Sigurs and colleagues[27,32–34] prospectively followed 46 children from infancy until the age of 18 years. Compared with 92 age-matched control subjects, exposure to RSV was associated with a significantly higher prevalence of asthma (39% in RSV-exposed vs 9% in controls), allergic rhinoconjunctivitis at age 13[27] (39% in RSV-exposed vs 15% in controls), and sensitization to allergens by age 18[34] (41% in RSV-exposed vs 14% in controls). The occurrence of RSV-induced bronchiolitis within the first year of life was associated with the development of asthma at ages 7 and 13 years. A 2-year prospective study conducted in Finland using PCR detection methods identified RSV, HRV, and other viruses as the major etiologic agents in acute expiratory wheeze in 293 hospitalized children, from 3 months to16 years of age.[35] Among the cases of acute expiratory wheezing, 88% involved a single respiratory virus while coinfection with several different viruses comprised 19% of all cases. The study found noticeable age-dependent variations in viral agent prevalence: RSV infects children younger than 11 months more than other age groups, whereas enteroviruses and HRV are most prevalent in children aged 12 months or older.[35] Unfortunately, no screening for atypical bacteria was performed to assess the prevalence of *C pneumoniae* or *M pneumoniae*.

In contrast, the 1980–1984 Tucson Children's Respiratory Study conducted by Stein and colleagues[31] and Taussig and colleagues[36] found RSV-associated LRI wheezing episodes by age 2 as an independent risk factor for wheezing and asthma at age 11 but not at age 13 years. Differences between the Swedish and Tucson study designs may account for the discrepancy in results at age 13 years. The Tucson questionnaire study enrolled healthy children in the first year of life, whereas the Swedish study investigated primarily infants younger than 6 months, who were hospitalized for RSV-induced bronchiolitis. Consequently, the Swedish study examined incidences of severe RSV-induced respiratory illnesses that resulted in enhanced airway obstruction and limited airway function. Furthermore, the Tucson study used immunofluorescence and viral culturing without PCR, and this may have resulted in missed detection of viral pathogens. For example, children who acquired virus-negative LRI before the age of 3 years were found to have an increased risk of frequent wheeze at age 8 compared with healthy controls[31]; moreover, LRIs caused by other agents, including rhinovirus, contributed a low proportion (14.4%) of the 472 reported LRIs and were not statistically correlated with frequent wheeze after age 3 years. These findings conflict with studies that identified HRV as the predominant cause of wheezy LRI in children in the age range of 6 to 17 years[8,26,30,37] or reports that found relatively low PCR detection of the atypical respiratory bacteria, *C pneumoniae* and *M pneumoniae*, in children.[15,38] Despite the design differences, the Sweden, Finland, and Tucson clinical studies all implicate RSV as an important pathogen in the subsequent development of early childhood asthma.

ETIOLOGIC AGENTS OF RESPIRATORY TRACT INFECTIONS

HRVs cause common colds and ARIs in both adults and children. HRVs are related to enteroviruses, such as poliovirus, echovirus, and Coxsackievirus. The positive-sense, single-stranded RNA genome of HRV is encased within a highly variable protein capsid composed of an icosahedral arrangement of 60 copies of viral proteins VP1, VP2, VP3, and VP4. Canyon-like depressions circle the vertices made of 5 triangular repeats of VP1,[39] and binding of the virus to cell receptors occurs near the canyons.[40]

Table 2
Clinical studies investigating respiratory tract infections in children

Location	Study Period	Population Studied	Detection Method	Pathogens Identified	Summary of Results
Edinburgh, UK[18]	Prospective cohort; Nov 1971–Oct 1974	360 children with acute wheezy bronchitis; >1 y old, first and readmissions	NPA for viral culture	HRV, HCoV, RSV, HPIV, IF, echovirus, Coxsackievirus, mumps	RV (16/38) and RSV (6/38) positive from 267 virus isolations
Wiltshire, UK[17,19,23]	Prospective cohort; Oct 1974–Apr 1976	72 episodes of wheezy bronchitis among 22 children (5–15 y)	Throat/sputum swabs for viral culture	HRV, IF, HPIV, RSV, AdV, M pneumoniae, coinfections	49% of episodes were virus-positive, predominantly RV
Turku, Finland[21]	Prospective cohort; Sep 1985–Aug 1986; Jan 1987	54 asthmatic children (1–6 y) with recurrent wheezy bronchitis	NPA for viral culture, serology	HCoV, HRV, AdV, IF, HPIV, M pneumoniae, coinfections	45% episodes positive for virus or M pneumoniae; predominantly HCoV outbreak of coronavirus
Southampton, UK[26]	Prospective cohort; Apr 1989–May 1990	108 children (9–11 y) reporting wheeze or cough	NPA for IF, viral culture, serology, reverse transcription (RT)-PCR, probes	HRV, HCoV, IF, HPIV, RSV, others	77% detected viral positive in 292 reported episodes & RV representing 2/3; 81% LRI
Nord-Pas de Calais, France[37]	Prospective cohort; Oct 1998–June 1999	113 children (2–16 y) with acute or active asthma	Nasal swabs for IF and RT-PCR, serology	HRV, RSV, AdV, HPIV, HCoV, enterovirus, C pneumoniae. M pneumoniae	RV (12%) and RSV (7.3%) of total of 38% virus-positive; 10% atypical bacteria-positive

Finland[35]	Prospective clinical trial	293 hospitalized children (3 mo to 16 y) for acute wheezing	PCR detection	HRV, RSV, enterovirus	HRV or RSV attributed to 88% cases; 19% cases from coinfections
Sweden[27,32-34]	Prospective cohort; Dec 1989–2009	46 children (<1–18 y); 92 age-matched healthy controls	PCR and culture	RSV	RSV-exposed subjects had 39% of asthma compared with unexposed (9%)
Atlanta, USA[8]	Case-control; Mar 2003–Feb 2004	142 enrolled children (2 groups: <6 or 6–17 y); 65 acute asthma cases and 77 well-controlled asthma controls	Nasal and throat swabs for PCR and RT-PCR	HRV, RSV, HMPV, HCoV, bocavirus, AdV, IF, HPIV, enterovirus	63.1% positive ≥ 1 viruses in case vs 23.4% in controls; predominantly RV
Perth, Australia[7,29]	Prospective cohort; Jul 1996–Jul 1999	236 atopic children enrolled, 198 children (<1–5 y)	NPA for PCR	HRV, HPIV, HMPV, RSV, HCoV, AdV, M pneumoniae, C pneumoniae, coinfections	69% ARI are virus-associated; predominantly RV (48.3%) and RSV (10.9%)
Madison, USA[30]	Prospective cohort; Sep 1998–current	259 children enrolled in COAST	NPA for PCR	HRV, RSV	90% of children with wheezy HRV-induced illness by 3 y subsequently acquired asthma at age 6 y

HRV-A and HRV-B diversity exceeds 100 serotypes, most of which were identified before the 1970s and continue to circulate, suggesting that emerging strains may not be new but rather previously unrecognized.[41] Highly sensitive genome sequencing and reverse transcription (RT)-PCR has generally replaced serotyping in diagnostics,[42–44] and researchers using this method discovered a third viral subgroup in 2006 called HRV-C that is associated with fall and winter asthma flares in children.[45,46]

Infecting mostly adults and children older than 3 years,[35] HRV enters through the upper respiratory tract via aerosolized droplets or transmission by hand contact.[47] HRV illnesses are usually noticeable within the first 3 days, accompanied by symptoms of the common cold, including nasal congestion, cough, sneezing, headaches, and sore throat.[48] Replication in epithelial cells occurs optimally at temperatures from 33° to 35°C, which lead investigators to consider HRV exclusively as an etiologic agent of upper RIs. Recent evidence, however, indicates that HRV is equally as important as a lower respiratory tract pathogen.[6,7] Symptoms of HRV infection often persist in the lower airways of adults[49] and the elderly,[50] yet evidence supporting the hypothesis that HRV causes chronic infections is limited because early longitudinal studies failed to identify HRV serotypes. Therefore, it is still unclear whether persistent HRV-induced ARIs result from chronic or new infections with different serotypes.[51] In support of the argument that HRVs do not cause chronic infections, a follow-up evaluation of the COAST study participants found consecutive, recurrent HRV infections with the same serotype to be uncommon.[52] Because a large number of serotypes recirculate in populations, reinfection with the same serotype is unlikely. Similar to other highly diverse viral pathogens, antigenic diversity could serve as a means for evading adaptive immunity.[51]

Despite differences in nucleotide sequence, antiviral drug susceptibility,[53,54] and capsid protein coding, nearly 90% of the HRV serotypes share a common cellular receptor for viral attachment to human epithelial cells.[55,56] Virus-cell surface attachment and subsequent infection is mediated through binding to intercellular adhesion molecule-1 (ICAM-1). ICAM-1 usually functions in leukocyte migration and antigen-independent adhesion for lymphocyte interaction.[57] ICAM-1 is the predominant receptor used by circulating HRV serotypes, and receptor compatibility appears to limit HRV host range.[58] ICAM-1 receptor is becoming recognized more and more as the attachment molecule of other pathogens, including rhinovirus,[39] some Coxsackie virus species,[59] and more recently, RSV.[60] Some evidence suggests that ICAM-1 expression is modulated by HRV after infection, making ICAM-1 a promising target for antiviral therapies.[61,62]

RSV is a member of the *Paramyxoviridae* family and is related to the etiologic agents of mumps, measles, and parainfluenza. As one of the leading causes of pediatric and geriatric respiratory diseases, RSV infections recur throughout life, and long-term immunity through vaccination has thus far been unsuccessful.[63,64] RSV infections result in approximately 10,000 deaths annually in persons older than 65 years and account for an estimated 30% of respiratory-related health care visits.[65] RSV mortality and morbidity increase among infants, the immunocompromised, and pulmonary hypertensive populations.[66,67] Seniors in particular remain at high risk for RSV infections because they may be exposed to nosocomial infections in the hospital or long-term care facilities.[68,69] The most notorious RSV vaccine failure used formalin-inactivated RSV (FI-RSV) to stimulate immunity, much like the Salk polio vaccine. Unfortunately, FI-RSV failed to elicit neutralizing antibody maturation[70] and in its place, CD4+ T-cell–mediated immunopathology was enhanced.[71,72]

At present, 2 prophylactic neutralizing antibodies against the RSV glycoprotein G have been reviewed by the Food and Drug Administration (FDA) and are available to high-risk infants,[64] but no effective vaccine or therapy is available for general populations. RSV disease onset resembles HRV infection with fever and wheezing. Several RSV proteins have been credited with suppression of the antiviral response, including nonstructural proteins 1 and 2 (NS1 and NS2), which disrupt JAK-STAT signaling and interferon (IFN)-β expression.[73,74] As a result, human RSV is a poor inducer of the antiviral type-1 IFN response. Primary and subsequent RSV infections lead to epithelial damage, lymphocyte infiltration, and airway inflammation.[75,76]

The single-stranded, negative-sense RNA genome of RSV is associated with a ribonucleoprotein (RNP) complex consisting of the nucleocapsid (N), phosphoprotein (P), and large (L) RNA-dependent RNA polymerase. On virion assembly and filamentous budding from infected epithelial cells, a bilipid envelope layer is derived from the host cell and interacts with the matrix (M) protein to surround the RNP.[77] A visual hallmark of RSV infections in monolayer culture cells is the formation of syncytia, which resemble multinucleated cells. Fusion of neighboring cells is initiated by RSV glycoproteins F and G and the small hydrophobic protein (SH), as plasmid transfection of these 3 viral proteins was found sufficient for syncytium formation.[78] F and G have numerous roles in disrupting host-cell responses to infection and interfering with antiviral signaling.[79] Investigations of individual RSV proteins provide evidence that RSV has the capacity to alter the host immune response and stimulate chronic inflammatory responses.

Viruses are not the only respiratory pathogens that can cause chronic infection and contribute to asthma. Although less prominent than the reports about HRV or RSV, longitudinal studies examining asthma exacerbations consistently recover and detect by PCR[15] the atypical bacteria, *Chlamydophila pneumoniae*[80,81] and *Mycobacterium pneumoniae*.[82] *C pneumoniae*, an etiologic agent of atypical pneumonia, is detectable by serology, culture, antigen detection, and complement fixation, and is found in 2% to 11% of cases of acute exacerbation in children.[7,15,37,83] Infections with *C pneumoniae* have been reported as high as 86% in adults when PCR detection was used.[9] Similarly, *M pneumoniae* contributes to 5.7% to 28.4% of pneumonia infections and is the predominant cause of tracheobronchitis.[84] As likely agents of chronic respiratory infection, *C pneumoniae* and *M pneumoniae* have been found to possess numerous mechanisms for disrupting innate, humoral, and cell-mediated immune responses.

MECHANISMS OF VIRUS-INDUCED IMMUNOPATHOLOGY AND ASTHMA EXACERBATIONS
Cellular Responses

Most HRV serotypes and RSV strains cause little cellular injury to bronchial epithelial cells in culture compared with infections with influenza A virus.[85,86] Some epithelial cell necrosis occurs and cellular debris accumulates in severe RSV infections,[87] but the majority of HRV- and RSV-induced pathology is attributed to indirect stimulation of host innate and adaptive immune cells. In vitro culture assays and animal model systems have been vital resources for studying disease pathogenesis. Unfortunately, primate cells are selectively permissive to a large number of HRV serotypes. Cells from rodents and other mammals lack the primate ICAM-1 receptor for HRV absorption and thus do not support the replication of the 90% of serotypes defined as the major group.[58] This problem has hindered studies of major-group HRV in vivo using animal models. Rodent cells are semipermissive to the remaining 10% (minor-group). Consequently, a minor-type rhinovirus-1B strain was used to develop rhinovirus 1B-induced asthma exacerbations in BALB/c mice.[88] Because RSV infections are relatively inefficient in adult rodents, high viral loads of RSV (10^5–10^7 pfu) are required to produce pathologic changes through intranasal[89–91] or intratracheal[87] inoculation. Despite some limitations, the murine models of virus-induced asthma exacerbation have provided a great deal of information regarding HRV and RSV pathogenesis.

Bronchoalveolar lavage (BAL) fluid recovered from minor-group RV1B HRV-infected mice often demonstrates neutrophilia, up-regulation of interleukin (IL)-6, IL-1β, RANTES (regulated on activation, normal T-cell expressed and secreted), and macrophage inflammatory protein-2 (MIP-2), and have increased production of T-cell chemokines within the first 2 days after infection.[86,88,92,93] Other chemokines elevated in murine RSV infection include monocyte chemoattractant protein (MCP-1), MIP-1α, interferon-inducible protein 10 (IP-10), IFN-γ, IL-5, and keratinocyte cytokine (KC).[87,94,95] The early flux of chemokines after HRV or RSV infection in mice is thought to contribute to lymphocyte activation and recruitment of neutrophils, macrophages, and eosinophils.

Translating the mouse studies to human subjects, Gern and colleagues and other groups[96–99] have recruited human patients, inoculated them with major-group rhinovirus-16 (RV16), and observed cellular responses to HRV infections. Surprisingly, cellular profiles after RV16 inoculation do not differ greatly among atopic asthmatics or nonatopic subjects.[100] Neutrophils were found to be the predominant cells recovered in BAL fluid,[97] but the neutrophilia was present in both groups during acute cold illnesses. No significant group-specific differences were observed in peak nasal viral titers or cold symptom scores. Bronchial biopsies from HRV-infected asthma patients display T-cell infiltration at the site of infection,[101] yet similar infiltration was absent in HRV-infected subjects without asthma.[99] Gern and colleagues[97,100,102] also observed elevated secretion of the neutrophil chemotaxin, IL-8, granulocyte colony-stimulating factor (G-CSF), IP-10, and MIP-2 in the sputum samples of infected asthma patients. Neutrophil recruitment was correlated with virus-mediated influx of IL-8[103] in both asthmatic and nonatopic individuals. Overall, the lack of cellular differences suggests that RV16 replication is not enhanced in atopic or asthmatic individuals.

The levels of eosinophil in sputum were significantly higher in asthmatics at baseline (7 or 14 days before inoculation) and in nasal lavage fluid during acute RV16 infection and following convalescence.[100] Although eosinophils are frequently elevated in nonatopic asthma patients as compared with healthy control groups without asthma,[104] eosinophils have been observed to persist in the lower airway of asthma subjects during the convalescence stage of RV16 infection[101]; a similar eosinophil persistence was not apparent in healthy individuals. Asthmatics had significantly increased secretion of MCP-1 in nasal lavage fluid at baseline (47%) compared with healthy controls (12%). Cumulatively, in vitro and in vivo studies identified some specific characteristics of virus-induced asthma exacerbation, including airway T-cell infiltration, virus-induced recruitment of neutrophils, and enhanced eosinophilia in the airway after recovery from rhinovirus infections.

Unlike HRV (particularly RV16), experimental infections with RSV have not been conducted extensively in human subjects. As of June 2010, only 2 reports used good manufacturing practice–quality wild-type RSV A2 in human experimental infections.[105,106] Healthy young adults aged 18 to 45 years were inoculated through nostril instillation with either a high (4.7 $\log_{10}$ tissue culture infective dose [$TCID_{50}$]) or a low (3.7 $\log_{10}$ $TCID_{50}$) RSV dose, and observed for 28 days. While neither control nor inoculated subjects demonstrated severe illness symptoms or lower respiratory disease with cough, shortness of breath, or wheezing, the 8 subjects given high doses and the 5 subjects given low doses shed virus for 1 to 8 days after inoculation.[105] Inoculated individuals exhibited mild systemic illness, with fever, chills, and fatigue, but respiratory symptoms remained localized to the upper respiratory tract. The study specifically measured viral titers and levels of viral proteins F and G, but did not report infiltrating cell profiles; thus, cellularity associated with experimental RSV A2 inoculation in humans was not directly comparable with that in murine or in vitro studies. Nasal and bronchial lavages from earlier clinical studies provide evidence that the infiltrating cell and chemokine profiles of RSV-infected patients are similar to those in HRV-infected murine models and human subjects.[93] Neutrophils are abundant in the nasal lavages of RSV-infected adults and infants[107] and in response to RSV infection, early cytokines and chemokines, like IL-12, IL-18, MIP-1α, IL-8, and RANTES, are up-regulated in the upper respiratory tract.[87,108–112] Lastly, detectable levels of eosinophils and factors associated with eosinophilic airway inflammation, such as eosinophil cationic protein and eotaxin, were observed to be highest among infants with RSV bronchiolitis when compared with control and non-RSV bronchiolitis.[113]

The significance of eosinophils in virus-induced asthma is widely debated, because eosinophils are often prevalent in areas of epithelial damage[104,114,115] and likely contribute to eosinophilic inflammation.[116,117] Conversely, observations from murine models demonstrate a protective role for eosinophils[118] in viral clearance through secretion of ribonucleases and other antiviral factors.[119] Eosinophil degranulation and release of eosinophil peroxidase (EPO) have been shown in vitro to be enhanced by the presence of viruses in coculture experiments with antigen-presenting cells (APCs; macrophage or dendritic cells) and CD4+ T cells.[120] Davoine and colleagues[120] demonstrated that the addition of HRV, RSV, or HPIV resulted in elevated EPO and/or leukotriene release. In addition, HRV and RSV stimulated production of IFN-γ in the presence of dendritic cells and T cells when eosinophils were absent. Other reports suggest that eosinophilia and secretion of eosinophil cationic protein (ECP) or RANTES are potential predictors of asthma and disease severity[121–123]; consequently, virus-induced eosinophilia may play a significant role in asthma exacerbations.

Molecular Mechanisms

RSV has been observed to exacerbate pulmonary stress in immunocompromised individuals by increasing airway resistance and potentiating hypoxemia.[124] RSV infections alter cytokine production and can result in chronic inflammation, respiratory failure, and death.[68,125] Cellular immunodeficiencies vary with age, and in persons older than 65 years, an alarming 78% of respiratory and pulmonary deaths are RSV-associated.[65,126] RSV employs multiple defenses against the innate and adaptive antiviral response,[110,127–129] and has the capacity to alter allergic responses and interfere with lymphocyte activation. RSV-infected infants have suppressed IFN-γ production and elevated IL-4, which are sufficient to stimulate IgE and T-helper 2 (Th2)-humoral responses.[130] Disruption of Type-I IFN responses through NS1, NS2, G and F, and other RSV proteins promotes viral replication and survival.[79]

Preliminary studies showed that IRF1 translocates to the nucleus and that the relative expression of IRF1, IRF3, and IRF7 was enhanced through silencing of NS1 with small-interfering RNA against NS1 in RSV-infected A549 lung adenocarcinoma epithelial cells.[75] IRF1 is important in apoptosis and activates T-helper 1 (Th1) responses while suppressing inappropriate Th2 responses.[131] IFN-regulatory factors have been shown to regulate T-cell differentiation,[132] and type-1 IFNs influence dendritic cell maturation[133] and Th1/Th2 cytokine production. Impairment of type-1 IFN or IRF1 expression and subsequent Th1 differentiation could result in a Th2-like inflammatory disease.[134,135] Alternatively, the RSV G protein may disrupt the Th1/Th2 cytokine balance. The secreted form of G (sG) contains a domain that mimics the chemokine CX3C[136] and induces production of IL-5 and IL-13, leading to eosinophilia through a mechanism that does not require IL-4.[137] Further examination is needed to determine the role of the G protein in inflammatory disease and Th2 responses. Collectively, the antagonistic RSV proteins give RSV the capacity to directly or indirectly impair immune cell activation and skew Th1/Th2 profiles.[138]

Rhinovirus infections trigger a cascade of events that lead to overproduction of mucus,[139] activation of nuclear factor (NF)-κB, and up-regulation of chemokines and cytokines.[86] In particular, a potent proinflammatory cytokine, tumor necrosis factor α (TNF-α), is produced by macrophages on NF-κB activation in RV16-infected macrophages derived from either THP-1 or primary monocytes.[140] NF-κB activation has been correlated with another respiratory virus, Sendai parainfluenza virus 1, which was used to model virus-induced asthma exacerbations in brown Norway rats.[141] Infection with Sendai virus substantially increased expression of the p50 subunit of NF-κB, implying functional activation of NF-κB.[142] On virus infection, respiratory epithelial cells show increased expression of several pattern recognition receptors (PRRs), including Toll-like receptors TLR3[143] and TLR4,[144] in response to HRV and RSV, respectively. RSV-mediated TLR4 overexpression was associated with sensitization of epithelial cells, resulting in enhanced IL-6 and IL-8 production after stimulation with bacterial lipopolysaccharide.[145] Lastly, both HRV and RSV use ICAM-1 as a receptor for viral attachment, and up-regulation of ICAM-1 could enhance viral infection. HRV has been observed to selectively enhance membrane-bound ICAM-1 while suppressing expression of secreted ICAM-1.[62] In recognition of this binding requirement for effective viral infection by either HRV or RSV, therapeutic applications have attempted to target ICAM-1 with blocking monoclonal antibodies.[146] Application of the ICAM-1 blocking antibody CFY196 showed promise in HRV infections, and reduced RV infection symptoms and length of disease in human subjects.[147–149] Similarly, blockage of ICAM-1 through a neutralizing monoclonal antibody to ICAM-1 attenuated RSV infection of epithelial cells in vitro.[60]

Similar to RSV infections, HRV infections often result in a reduction in the IFN-γ/IL-5 mRNA ratio, as seen in the experimental RV16 infection of human subjects.[98] Relatively weak Th1-like responses were also attributed to more severe respiratory disease and longer viral shedding. In human trials, asthmatic individuals did not have increased risk of HRV infection. Instead, the symptoms of clinical illness extended for longer times and were reported as more severe than in healthy, nonasthmatic cohabiting partners who had acquired HRV infections.[6] Whereas healthy controls usually had mild URI for 3 days, asthma patients developed both upper and lower respiratory tract symptoms for up to 5 days. A distortion of Th1/Th2 responses is expected to predispose subjects to more severe allergic reactions.[93,138,150] HRV infections in vitro stimulate IL-4 up-regulation in the peripheral blood mononuclear cells (PBMCs) of atopic asthmatics,[151] which contrasts with the usually observed decrease in IL-4 in PBMCs of healthy controls. Likewise, after RSV infection, ovalbumin-allergic mice have airway hyperresponsiveness and enhanced Th2 responses, accompanied by an up-regulation of IL-4 and increased eosinophilia in the lungs, on inhalation of ovalbumin.[152]

HRV has also been demonstrated to attenuate the type-1 IFN response through disruption of IRF3 activation.[153] Although the mechanism may be different, RV14 infection in A549 decreased the nuclear translocation of IRF3 as compared with cells infected with vesicular stomatitis virus (VSV), which is known to induce IFN-β responses. Moreover, immunoblots displayed a loss in the homodimer form of IRF3 in RV14-infected cells compared with VSV-infected cells at both 4 hours and 7 hours after infection. Of note, the expression of PRR-like melanoma differentiation-associated gene 5 (MDA5) or mitochondrial antiviral signaling (MAVS) protein were unchanged in lysates after infection with RV14 at 4 or 7 hours after infection. Together, this evidence suggests that RV14 disrupts nuclear translocation of IRF3 and suppresses IFN-β production after infection without disrupting either MDA5 or MAVS. **Fig. 1** illustrates the mechanisms by which RSV and HRV infections may skew the Th1/Th2 profiles and enhance Th2 responses in allergic or asthmatic individuals.

THERAPEUTIC APPROACHES TO RESPIRATORY VIRAL INFECTIONS

Developing efficacious and cost-effective antivirals against HRV and RSV has proven to be a continuing challenge for researchers and clinicians (**Table 3**). HRV capsid surface proteins are highly variable among the 100+ serotypes, and passive immunization will likely provide marginal, if any, protection. Because most HRV-induced illnesses in healthy individuals do not lead to hospitalizations, with cold-like symptoms peaking within 2 to 3 days and usually subsiding within a week, therapeutic benefits of any HRV intervention would need to significantly outweigh the risks associated from delivering treatment or immunizing with a vaccine. As with the failed clinical trials of FI-RSV, the associated dangers from vaccine delivery are unpredictable and could result in symptoms that are more serious. Conversely, if respiratory viral agents contribute to the development of asthma, prophylactic use of antivirals has the potential to prevent ARI as well as the chronic illness. Current antiviral drugs target the steps involved in viral propagation to suppress the spread of infection,[64,154] including attachment, replication, protein synthesis, and release of viral progeny, as illustrated in **Fig. 2**. Alternatively, supplementation with IFNs promotes antiviral and immunologic effects, thereby decreasing cell susceptibility; intranasal IFN has demonstrated effective prophylactic potential in enterovirus and HRV studies.[154] In an RSV-infected murine model, intranasal administration of the plasmid encoding IFN-γ decreased the neutrophilia and pulmonary inflammation that is associated with RSV-induced disease.[155]

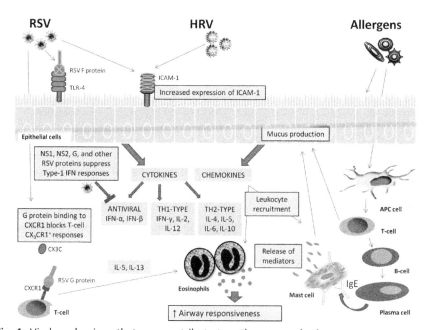

Fig. 1. Viral mechanisms that may contribute to asthma exacerbations.

Table 3
Experimental antiviral pharmacologic agents for HRV and RSV infections

Compound Class	Virus Infection	Examples	Current Status
Antibodies to host receptors	RSV and HRV	Monoclonal antibodies to ICAM-1	HRV infections reduced by >90%[148]; reduced RSV infections in human epithelial cells[60]
Small-molecule fusion inhibitors	RSV	BMS-433771, RFI-641	Prophylactic oral administration reduced lungs viral titers in RSV-infected mice; however, postinfection delivery failed to decrease virus infection.[180] Phase 1/2 clinical trials discontinued[181]
Attachment inhibitor; specific for G glycoprotein	RSV	MBX-300 (NMSO3)	Effective in vitro and in vivo, with EC_{50} 53 value times lower than that of ribavirin.[162] Clinical trials expected
Peptide-based antisense agents	HRV and enteroviruses	PPMO (peptide-conjugated phosphorodiamidate morpholino oligomers)	~80% higher survival rates in rodent HRV-infected models as compared with untreated controls[163]
Small-molecule inhibitor of L-protein	RSV	YM-53403	RSV-specific inhibition of viral RNA replication[164]
siRNA	RSV	NS1	Delivery of nanoparticles with siRNA against NS1 significantly attenuated RSV infection in rodent models[75,182]

Several promising antiviral agents physically disrupt the interaction between the virion and host-cell receptor.[156–158] In theory, this will prevent attachment of the virus or reduce its ability to fuse with and infect the cell. The humanized monoclonal antibody against the RSV F protein, palivizumab, is currently the only pharmacologic agent that is FDA-approved for administration to high-risk infants for preventing severe LRI.[159,160] **Table 4** summarizes other viral targets and antiviral compounds, such as protease or viral protein inhibitors, which have undergone or are undergoing clinical studies for potential therapeutic applications in humans. Recent clinical trials have eliminated several promising but inadequate and ineffective antiviral candidates. For example, the protease inhibitor rupintrivir demonstrated prophylactic efficacy and reduced viral load in experimental HRV infection[158] but failed to protect against natural HRV infection.[161] As a result, no future clinical applications are being pursued.

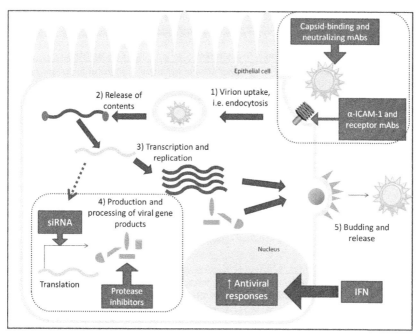

Fig. 2. Targets for antivirals against RSV and HRV.

Despite the disappointments with FI-RSV vaccine and rupintrivir, alternative antiviral strategies are being investigated, including the use of large chemical-library screening for identifying specific, small-molecule inhibitors and the delivery of small-interfering RNA to silence viral protein gene expression. As complementary pharmacologic agents or alternatives to passive immunization, small-molecule inhibitors and viral protein antagonists are showing promise in tissue-culture and animal models.[75,162–164] A few of these alternative, experimental studies are proceeding to clinical application and may be successful. DeVincenzo and colleagues,[106] in 2010, were the first group to demonstrate a proof-of-concept application of RNAi (RNA interference) for protection against RSV by delivering siRNA to the respiratory tract in human subjects given experimental RSV infection. RNAi-based therapies have shown promise in vitro and in animal models for various human diseases, predominantly cancer. In rodent models, intranasal delivery of siRNA against the nucleocapsid (N) protein (ALN-RSV01) before or 1 to 2 days after RSV inoculation reduced lung viral titer loads by at least 2 logs.[165] Gene silencing of the well-conserved RSV N protein disrupts viral replication through impairment of the RSV RNA polymerase. ALN-RSV01 is the first siRNA delivered to humans via the intranasal route for specifically combating a microbial pathogen.[165] In a randomized, phase 2 study conducted by DeVincenzo and colleagues,[106] ALN-RSV01 decreased RSV infection in experimentally RSV-inoculated subjects by 38% compared with placebo-treated controls, as diagnosed by 2 culture-based assays. From days 4 to 7 after infection, the mean viral load in pfu/mL decreased approximately 1 log as detected by quantitative RT-PCR. The antiviral effect of ALN-RSV01 was found to be independent of preexisting RSV-neutralizing antibodies or cytokine concentrations. Thus, ALN-RSV01 exhibits potential for therapeutic use in healthy adults. However, low statistical power and insufficient sample numbers hinder the study's reliability in evaluating the antiviral dose-responsiveness of ALN-RSV01 with respect to viral load and disease symptoms

Table 4
Clinical trials of HRV and RSV antiviral pharmacologic agents

Compound Class	Virus Infection	Examples	Current Status
Antibodies to glycoproteins	RSV	Monoclonal antibody to F protein (Palivizumab)	Multicenter, phase 3 clinical trial in 1997; reduced length of RSV hospitalization, disease severity, and admission to intensive care unit[160]
Antibodies to host receptors	HRV and potentially RSV	Soluble ICAM-1 (Tremacamra)	Four randomized clinical trials in 1996; marginal effectiveness within 12 h of experimental infection with HRV39[156]
Antibodies to glycoproteins	RSV	Monoclonal antibody to F protein (Motavizumab)	Currently undergoing phase 2 and phase 2 clinical studies; pending FDA review as of Aug 2010[157]
Capsid-function inhibitor	HRV and enteroviruses	Binds to capsid and disrupts uncoating (Pleconaril)	Phase 2 clinical trial in 2006; results unreleased Two phase 2 clinical trials in 2003 showed reduced cold symptoms and shorter duration of cold[158]
Protease inhibitors	HRV and enteroviruses	Irreversible inhibitor of HRV 3C protease (Rupintrivir)	Phase 2 clinical studies in 2003; reduced viral load after experimental infection with HRV39[177] but not with natural infections[161]
Protease inhibitors	HRV and enteroviruses	Irreversible inhibitor of HRV 3C protease (Compound I)	Phase 1 clinical studies completed in 2003; reduced viral loads[161,178] but no future trials pending
N-protein inhibitor	RSV	RSV-604	Phase 1 in 2006, phase 2 ongoing[179]
Antisense to N protein	RSV	ALN-RSV01	Phase 1 in 2007, phase 2 trial in 2009. First siRNA delivery to respiratory tract[106,165]

over the entire term of the study. ALN-RSV01 remains an attractive antiviral candidate because few adverse affects were observed in normal adult humans. Further investigations are needed to test the efficacy of RNAi against natural infections, and its applicability to infants and RSV risk groups.

POSTINFECTION THERAPEUTICS WITH ANTI-INFLAMMATORY AGENTS

HRV and RSV are highly infectious and ubiquitous respiratory pathogens, but eradication of either species in the near future is highly unlikely. To cope with virus-induced bronchiolitis, a variety of anti-inflammatory pharmacologic agents, such as broncho-dilators and steroids, are recommended for susceptible individuals to reduce airway inflammation. National health organization guidelines often recommend inhaled corti-costeroids (ICS) as the primary treatment for recurrent asthma, followed by short- or long-acting β2-agonists (SABA and LABA) and cysteinyl-leukotriene (Cys-LT) receptor agonists (LTRA).[166,167] ICS act to reduce asthma symptoms, and help improve forced expiratory volume in 1 second (FEV_1) and peak expiratory flow rate (PEFR).[168] Although ICS demonstrate potency against other inflammatory diseases and continue to be the preferred drug for managing asthma symptoms, evidence is lacking to support ICS in preventing virus-induced wheezing in corticosteroid-unresponsive subpopulations.[168,169] In a clinical study of United Kingdom children aged between 10 and 30 months hospitalized for wheezy ARI, oral corticosteroid prednisolone administration over 5 consecutive days failed to reduce disease severity or hospitali-zation length significantly.[169] According to a retrospective United States study, steroid insensitivity was frequent in adolescent populations (~14 years of age); up to 24% of patients with severe asthma failed to respond to glucocorticosteroid therapy.[170] Inconsistent responsiveness to ICS likely results from genetic variability, atopic family history, and airway fibrosis that accumulates after severe epithelial damage.[171] At present there is insufficient information to assess the effects of ICS on virus-induced illnesses.

While controversy over the efficacy of ICS on virus-induced ARI continues, recent clinical studies suggest leukotriene receptor antagonists may alleviate virus-induced bronchiolitis. Two clinical trials of the Cys-LT known as montelukast demonstrated efficacy against RSV-induced asthma exacerbations as compared with placebo. Bis-gaard and the Study Group on Montelukast and Respiratory Syncytial Virus[172] moni-tored children from 3 to 36 months old for 28 days to compare the effect of chewable tablets of montelukast on RSV-induced bronchiolitis, compared with placebo. In the randomized, double-blind, placebo-controlled study, subjects receiving montelukast reported fewer symptoms, and disease severity was significantly less than in the placebo-receiving control population. Post hoc analysis of a similar, but more exten-sive study by Bisgaard and colleagues[173] revealed a comparable therapeutic effect of montelukast on RSV bronchiolitis. Furthermore, Kim and colleagues[174] specifically investigated the anti-inflammatory effects of montelukast in infants for a 12-month period by analyzing eosinophil degranulation, as measured by the secretion of an eosinophil biomarker, eosinophil-derived neurotoxin (EDN). EDN is more stable than other eosinophil biomarkers and is therefore a better representation of eosinophil inflammatory activity than eosinophil counts alone. For that reason, the group used EDN levels for estimating disease severity and recurrent wheeze. Kim and colleagues observed significantly higher levels of EDN in RSV-infected populations than in unin-fected controls; furthermore, patients receiving a 3-month course of montelukast had significantly lower levels of EDN than the placebo-treated group. Based on this evidence, montelukast could be used to treat RSV bronchiolitis; however, further investigation is needed to understand the antiviral mechanism and how different subpopulations respond to the drug.

CHALLENGES AND OPPORTUNITIES FOR ASTHMA THERAPY

Although infections with other viruses and bacteria may play roles in wheezing, airway inflammation, and hyperactivity, HRV and RSV are the primary etiologic agents asso-ciated with acute respiratory illness and asthma exacerbations.[8,26] In 2006, 197 chil-dren hospitalized for asthma exacerbations and wheezing episodes were examined in a year-long prospective, cross-sectional study in Buenos Aires.[24] The ages ranged from 3 months to 16 years, and PCR was used for detecting virus and bacteria in nasopharyngeal aspirate samples. In agreement with others, Maffey and colleagues[24] found virus or bacteria in 78% of the cases (40% RSV, 4.5% HRV, 4.5% M pneumoniae, and 2% C pneumoniae). With increased sensitivity, PCR has enabled detection of pathogens that would otherwise be nondetectable by culture methods. In addition, the methods for recruiting, diagnosing, and examining ARI subjects are becoming standardized, allowing better comparisons with other studies. However, several factors continue to cause variability in community-based studies. Environmental, economic, and social variables will continue to challenge how diagnosticians and health care workers collect data. In some studies, obtaining controls is difficult due to semi-invasive procedures, and comparisons must often be made with asymptomatic individuals.[26] Furthermore, the statistical power of these studies is reduced by the relatively small number of eligible and cooperative participants. While most cohort investigations study infants and older children hospitalized for severe ARI symptoms, additional studies on less severe cases should be done to determine how mild RSV infections are associated with wheeze.

Despite the strong evidence for a link between asthma and respiratory infections, the direction of causality between viral infections and asthma is still heatedly debated. Although there is a growing body of evidence supporting a causal relationship for HRV, a similar relationship for RSV is difficult to prove because virtually all children have been infected with RSV by the age of 2 years[66,79]; therefore, the development of asthma likely depends on genetic and/or atopic factors.[175] Simões and colleagues[176] recently reported new evidence that associates RSV infection with the development of recurrent wheeze in nonatopic infants, in a worldwide, multicenter, 24-month investigation. Prophylactic delivery of palivizumab decreased the relative risk of recurrent wheezing in nonatopic infants by 80%. Surprisingly, palivizumab failed to improve wheezing outcomes in infants from families with atopic genetic backgrounds. As one of the first investigations to evaluate the protective effects of palivizumab against recurrent wheeze, the evidence from Simões and colleagues suggests that early-life RSV infection significantly predisposes nonatopic populations to recurrent wheeze. Additional investigations that use prophylaxis, including passive immunization through neutralizing antibodies and other antiviral candidates, are needed to better understand the contribution of viral infections to the development of asthma. Small-interfering RNA, neutralizing antibodies, and RSV fusion inhibitors show promise in vitro and in murine models, but the feasibility of broad-use application remains to be tested.[64] As the asthma epidemic persists and wheezing conditions continue to increase the costs of health care, the world awaits the application of more effective prophylactics to prevent microbe-associated respiratory illnesses.

REFERENCES

1. Bloom B, Cohen RA, Freeman G. Summary health statistics for U.S. children: National Health Interview Survey, 2008. Vital Health Stat 2009;10(244):55.
2. Akinbami L. NCHS Health E-Stat: asthma prevalence, health care use and mortality: United States, 2003-05. Hyattsville (MD): Office of Information Services; 2006.
3. National Heart, Lung and Blood Institute chartbook. Bethesda (MD): National Institute of Health U.S. Department of Health and Human Services; 2009.

4. Asher MI, Montefort S, Björkstén B, et al. Worldwide time trends in the prevalence of symptoms of asthma, allergic rhinoconjunctivitis, and eczema in childhood: ISAAC phases one and three repeat multicountry cross-sectional surveys. Lancet 2006;368(9537):733–43.

5. Moorman JE, Rudd RA, Johnson RA, et al. National surveillance for asthma—United States, 1980-2004. MMVR Surveill Summ 2007;56(SS8 Suppl S):1–54.

6. Corne JM, Marshall C, Smith S, et al. Frequency, severity, and duration of rhinovirus infections in asthmatic and non-asthmatic individuals: a longitudinal cohort study. Lancet 2002;359(9309):831–4

7. Merci MH, Nicholas HdK, Tatiana K, et al. Early-life respiratory viral infections, atopic sensitization, and risk of subsequent development of persistent asthma. J Allergy Clin Immunol 2007;119(5):1105–10.

8. Khetsuriani N, Kazerouni NN, Erdman DD, et al. Prevalence of viral respiratory tract infections in children with asthma. J Allergy Clin Immunol 2007;119(2):314–21.

9. Cosentini R, Tarsia P, Canetta C, et al. Severe asthma exacerbation: role of acute Chlamydophila pneumoniae and Mycoplasma pneumoniae infection. Respir Res 2008;9(1):48.

10. Stockton J, Ellis JS, Saville M, et al. Multiplex PCR for typing and subtyping influenza and respiratory syncytial viruses. J Clin Microbiol 1998;36(10):2990–5.

11. Loens K, Goossens H, de Laat C, et al. Detection of rhinoviruses by tissue culture and two independent amplification techniques, nucleic acid sequence-based amplification and reverse transcription-PCR, in children with acute respiratory infections during a winter season. J Clin Microbiol 2006;44(1):166–71.

12. Lau LT, Feng XY, Lam TY, et al. Development of multiplex nucleic acid sequence-based amplification for detection of human respiratory tract viruses. J Virol Methods 2010;168(1–2):251–4.

13. Kistler A, Avila PC, Rouskin S, et al. Pan-viral screening of respiratory tract infections in adults with and without asthma reveals unexpected human coronavirus and human rhinovirus diversity. J Infect Dis 2007;196(6):817–25.

14. Lambert HP, Stern H. Infective factors in exacerbations of bronchitis and asthma. Br Med J 1972;3(5822):323.

15. Freymuth F, Vabret A, Brouard J, et al. Detection of viral, Chlamydia pneumoniae and Mycoplasma pneumoniae infections in exacerbations of asthma in children. J Clin Virol 1999;13(3):131–9.

16. Buscho RO, Saxtan D, Shultz PS, et al. Infections with viruoco and Mycoplasma pneumoniae during exacerbations of chronic bronchitis. J Infect Dis 1978;137(4):377–83.

17. Horn ME, Reed SE, Taylor P. Role of viruses and bacteria in acute wheezy bronchitis in childhood—study of sputum. Arch Dis Child 1979;54(8):587–92.

18. Mitchell I, Inglis H, Simpson H. Viral-infection in wheezy bronchitis and asthma in children. Arch Dis Child 1976;51(9):707–11.

19. Horn ME, Gregg I. Role of viral infection and host factors in acute episodes of asthma and chronic bronchitis. Chest 1973;63(Suppl 4):44S–8S.

20. Sanders S, Norman AP. Bacterial flora of upper respiratory tract in children with severe asthma. J Allergy 1968;41(6):319.

21. Mertsola J, Ziegler T, Ruuskanen O, et al. Recurrent wheezy bronchitis and viral respiratory-infections. Arch Dis Child 1991;66(1):124–9.

22. Beasley R, Coleman ED, Hermon Y, et al. Viral respiratory-tract infection and exacerbations of asthma in adult patients. Thorax 1988;43(9):679–83.

23. Horn ME, Brain E, Gregg I, et al. Respiratory viral infection in childhood. A survey in general practice, Roehampton 1967-1972. J Hyg (Lond) 1975;74(2): 157–68.

24. Maffey AF, Barrero PR, Venialgo C, et al. Viruses and atypical bacteria associated with asthma exacerbations in hospitalized children. Pediatr Pulmonol 2010;45(6):619–25.

25. Wolf DG, Greenberg D, Kalkstein D, et al. Comparison of human metapneumovirus, respiratory syncytial virus and influenza A virus lower respiratory tract infections in hospitalized young children. Pediatr Infect Dis J 2006;25(4):320–4.

26. Johnston SL, Pattemore PK, Sanderson G, et al. Community study of role of viral infections in exacerbations of asthma in 9–11 year old children. BMJ 1995; 310(6989):1225–9.

27. Sigurs N, Gustafsson PM, Bjarnason R, et al. Severe respiratory syncytial virus bronchiolitis in infancy and asthma and allergy at age 13. Am J Respir Crit Care Med 2005;171(2):137–41.

28. Bush A. Practice imperfect—treatment for wheezing in preschoolers. N Engl J Med 2009;360(4):409–10.

29. Kusel MM, de Klerk NH, Holt PG, et al. Role of respiratory viruses in acute upper and lower respiratory tract illness in the first year of life—a birth cohort study. Pediatr Infect Dis J 2006;25(8):680–6.

30. Jackson DJ, Gangnon RE, Evans MD, et al. Wheezing rhinovirus illnesses in early life predict asthma development in high-risk children. Am J Respir Crit Care Med 2008;178(7):667–72.

31. Stein RT, Sherrill D, Morgan WJ, et al. Respiratory syncytial virus in early life and risk of wheeze and allergy by age 13 years. Lancet 1999;354(9178):541–5.

32. Sigurs N, Bjarnason R, Sigurbergsson F, et al. Asthma and immunoglobulin e antibodies after respiratory syncytial virus bronchiolitis: a prospective cohort study with matched controls. Pediatrics 1995;95(4):500–5.

33. Sigurs N, Bjarnason R, Sigurbergsson F, et al. Respiratory syncytial virus bronchiolitis in infancy is an important risk factor for asthma and allergy at age 7. Am J Respir Crit Care Med 2000;161(5):1501–7.

34. Sigurs N, Aljassim F, Kjellman B, et al. Asthma and allergy patterns over 18 years after severe RSV bronchiolitis in the first year of life. Thorax 2010. [Epub ahead of print].

35. Jartti T, Lehtinen P, Vuorinen T, et al. Respiratory picornaviruses and respiratory syncytial virus as causative agents of acute expiratory wheezing in children. Emerg Infect Dis 2004;10(6):1095–101.

36. Taussig LM, Wright AL, Morgan WJ, et al. The Tucson Children's Respiratory Study: I. Design and implementation of a prospective study of acute and chronic respiratory illness in children. Am J Epidemiol 1989;129(6):1219–31.

37. Thumerelle C, Deschildre A, Bouquillon C, et al. Role of viruses and atypical bacteria in exacerbations of asthma in hospitalized children: a prospective study in the Nord-Pas de Calais region (France). Pediatr Pulmonol 2003;35(2): 75–82.

38. Cunningham AF, Johnston SL, Julious SA, et al. Chronic Chlamydia pneumoniae infection and asthma exacerbations in children. Eur Respir J 1998;11(2):345–9.

39. Bella J, Rossmann MG. Review: rhinoviruses and their ICAM receptors. J Struct Biol 1999;128(1):69–74.

40. Colonno RJ, Condra JH, Mizutani S, et al. Evidence for the direct involvement of the rhinovirus canyon in receptor binding. Proc Natl Acad Sci U S A 1988; 85(15):5449–53.

41. Monto AS, Bryan ER, Ohmit S. Rhinovirus infections in Tecumseh, Michigan—frequency of illness and number of serotypes. J Infect Dis 1987;156(1):43–9.
42. Ann CP, Jennifer AR, Stephen BL. Analysis of the complete genome sequences of human rhinovirus. J Allergy Clin Immunol 2010;125(6):1190–9.
43. Kistler AL, Webster DR, Rouskin S, et al. Genome-wide diversity and selective pressure in the human rhinovirus. Virol J 2007;3(4):40.
44. Tapparel C, Junier T, Gerlach D, et al. New complete genome sequences of human rhinoviruses shed light on their phylogeny and genomic features. BMC Genomics 2007;10(8):224.
45. Lee WM, Kiesner C, Pappas T, et al. A diverse group of previously unrecognized human rhinoviruses are common causes of respiratory illnesses in infants. PLoS ONE 2007;2(10):e966.
46. Wos M, Sanak M, Soja J, et al. The presence of rhinovirus in lower airways of patients with bronchial asthma. Am J Respir Crit Care Med 2008;177(10):1082–9.
47. Gwaltney JM Jr, Hendley JO. Rhinovirus transmission: one if by air, two if by hand. Am J Epidemiol 1978;107(5):357–61.
48. Kelly JT, Busse WW. Host immune responses to rhinovirus: mechanisms in asthma. J Allergy Clin Immunol 2008;122(4):671–82.
49. Wos M, Sanak M, Burchell L, et al. Rhinovirus infection in lower airways of asthmatic patients. J Allergy Clin Immunol 2006;117(2 Suppl 1):S314.
50. Louie JK, Yagi S, Nelson FA, et al. Rhinovirus outbreak in a long term care facility for elderly persons associated with unusually high mortality. Clin Infect Dis 2005;41(2):262–5.
51. Regamey N, Kaiser L. Rhinovirus infections in infants: is respiratory syncytial virus ready for the challenge? Eur Respir J 2008;32(2):249–51.
52. Jartti T, Lee WM, Pappas T, et al. Serial viral infections in infants with recurrent respiratory illnesses. Eur Respir J 2008;32(2):314–20.
53. Ledford RM, Patel NR, Demenczuk TM, et al. VP1 sequencing of all human rhinovirus serotypes: insights into genus phylogeny and susceptibility to antiviral capsid-binding compounds. J Virol 2004;78(7):3663–74.
54. Graat JM, Schouten EG, Heijnen MLA, et al. A prospective, community-based study on virologic assessment among elderly people with and without symptoms of acute respiratory infection. J Clin Epidemiol 2003;56(12):1218–23.
55. Abraham G, Colonno RJ. Many rhinovirus serotypes share the same cellular receptor. J Virol 1984;51(2):340–5.
56. Greve JM, Davis G, Meyer AM, et al. The major human rhinovirus receptor is ICAM-1. Cell 1989;56(5):839–47.
57. vandeStolpe A, vanderSaag PT. Intercellular adhesion molecule-1. J Mol Med 1996;74(1):13–33.
58. Lomax NB, Yin FH. Evidence for the role of the p2-protein of human rhinovirus in its host range change. J Virol 1989;63(5):2396–9.
59. Xiao C, Bator-Kelly CM, Rieder E, et al. The crystal structure of Coxsackievirus A21 and its interaction with ICAM-1. Structure 2005;13(7):1019–33.
60. Behera AK, Matsuse H, Kumar M, et al. Blocking intercellular adhesion molecule-1 on human epithelial cells decreases respiratory syncytial virus infection. Biochem Biophys Res Commun 2001;280(1):188–95.
61. Grunberg K, Sharon RF, Hiltermann TJN, et al. Experimental rhinovirus 16 infection increases intercellular adhesion molecule-1 expression in bronchial epithelium of asthmatics regardless of inhaled steroid treatment. Clin Exp Allergy 2000;30(7):1015–23.

62. Whiteman SC, Bianco A, Knight RA, et al. Human rhinovirus selectively modulates membranous and soluble forms of its intercellular adhesion molecule-1 (ICAM-1) receptor to promote epithelial cell infectivity. J Biol Chem 2003; 278(14):11954–61.

63. Varga SM. Fixing a failed vaccine. Nat Med 2009;15(1):21–2.

64. Empey KM, Peebles RS Jr, Kolls JK. Reviews of anti-infective agents: pharmacologic advances in the treatment and prevention of respiratory syncytial virus. Clin Infect Dis 2010;50(9):1258–67.

65. Falsey AR, Hennessey PA, Formica MA, et al. Respiratory syncytial virus infection in elderly and high-risk adults. N Engl J Med 2005;352(17):1749–59.

66. Zhang W, Lockey RF, Mohapatra SS. Respiratory syncytial virus: immunopathology and control. Expert Rev Clin Immunol 2006;2(1):169–79.

67. Macdonald NE, Hall CB, Suffin SC, et al. Respiratory syncytial viral-infection in infants with congenital heart-disease. N Engl J Med 1982;307(7):397–400.

68. Johnstone J, Majumdar SR, Fox JD, et al. Viral infection in adults hospitalized with community-acquired pneumonia: prevalence, pathogens, and presentation. Chest 2008;134(6):1141–8.

69. Garcia R, Raad I, Abi-Said D, et al. Nosocomial respiratory syncytial virus infections: prevention and control in bone marrow transplant patients. Infect Control Hosp Epidemiol 1997;18(6):412–6.

70. Delgado MF, Coviello S, Monsalvo AC, et al. Lack of antibody affinity maturation due to poor Toll-like receptor stimulation leads to enhanced respiratory syncytial virus disease. Nat Med 2009;15(1):34–41.

71. Kim HW, Canchola JG, Brandt CD, et al. Respiratory syncytial virus disease in infants despite prior administration of antigenic inactivated vaccine. Am J Epidemiol 1969;89(4):422–34.

72. Connors M, Giese NA, Kulkarni AB, et al. Enhanced pulmonary histopathology induced by respiratory syncytial virus (RSV) challenge of formalin-inactivated RSV-immunized BALB/c mice is abrogated by depletion of interleukin-4 (IL-4) and IL-10. J Virol 1994;68(8):5321–5.

73. Spann KM, Tran KC, Collins PL. Effects of nonstructural proteins ns1 and ns2 of human respiratory syncytial virus on interferon regulatory factor 3, NF-{kappa}B, and pro-inflammatory cytokines. J. Virol. 2005;79(9):5353–62.

74. Lo MS, Brazas RM, Holtzman MJ. Respiratory syncytial virus nonstructural proteins ns1 and ns2 mediate inhibition of stat2 expression and alpha/beta interferon responsiveness. J Virol 2005;79(14):9315–9.

75. Zhang W, Yang H, Kong X, et al. Inhibition of respiratory syncytial virus infection with intranasal siRNA nanoparticles targeting the viral NS1 gene. Nat Med 2005; 11(1):56–62.

76. Kong X, Zhang W, Lockey RF, et al. Respiratory syncytial virus infection in Fischer 344 rats is attenuated by short interfering RNA against the RSV-NS1 gene. Genet Vaccines Ther 2007;5:4.

77. Takimoto T, Portner A. Molecular mechanism of paramyxovirus budding. Virus Res 2004;106(2):133–45.

78. Heminway BR, Yu Y, Tanaka Y, et al. Analysis of respiratory syncytial virus F-protein, G-protein, and SH-protein in cell-fusion. Virology 1994;200(2): 801–5.

79. Oshansky CM, Zhang W, Moore E, et al. The host response and molecular pathogenesis associated with respiratory syncytial virus infection. Future Microbiol 2009;4(3):279–97.

80. Hahn DL, Dodge RW, Golubjatnikov R. Association of *Chlamydia pneumoniae* (strain TWAR) infection with wheezing, asthmatic bronchitis, and adult-onset asthma. JAMA 1991;266(2):225–30.

81. Hahn D, Bukstein D, Luskin A, et al. Evidence for *Chlamydia pneumoniae* infection in steroid-dependent asthma. Ann Allergy Asthma Immunol 1998;80:45–9.

82. Kraft M, Cassell GH, Henson JE, et al. Detection of *Mycoplasma pneumoniae* in the airways of adults with chronic asthma. Am J Respir Crit Care Med 1998; 158(3):998–1001.

83. Allegra L, Blasi F, Centanni S, et al. Acute exacerbations of asthma in adults: role of *Chlamydia pneumoniae* infection. Eur Respir J 1994;7:2165–8.

84. Clyde WA. *Mycoplasma pneumoniae* respiratory-disease symposium—summation and significance. Yale J Biol Med 1983;56(5-6):523–7.

85. Zhang L, Peeples ME, Boucher RC, et al. Respiratory syncytial virus infection of human airway epithelial cells is polarized, specific to ciliated cells, and without obvious cytopathology. J Virol 2002;76(11):5654–66.

86. Schroth MK, Grimm E, Frindt P, et al. Rhinovirus replication causes RANTES production in primary bronchial epithelial cells. Am J Respir Cell Mol Biol 1999;20(6):1220–8.

87. Miller AL, Terry LB, Lukacs NW. Respiratory syncytial virus-induced chemokine production: linking viral replication to chemokine production in vitro and in vivo. J Infect Dis 2004;189(8):1419–30.

88. Bartlett NW, Walton RP, Edwards MR, et al. Mouse models of rhinovirus-induced disease and exacerbation of allergic airway inflammation. Nat Med 2008;14(2): 199–204.

89. Peebles RS Jr, Graham BS. Pathogenesis of respiratory syncytial virus infection in the murine model. Proc Am Thorac Soc 2005;2(2):110–5.

90. Mejias A, Chávez-Bueno S, Gómez AM, et al. Respiratory syncytial virus persistence: evidence in the mouse model. Pediatr Infect Dis J 2008;27(Suppl 10): S60–2.

91. Graham B, Perkins M, Wright P, et al. Primary respiratory syncytial virus infection in mice. J Med Virol 1988;26(2):153–62.

92. Bonville C, Rosenberg H, Domachowske J. Macrophage inflammatory protein-1alpha and RANTES are present in nasal secretions during ongoing upper respiratory tract infection. Pediatr Allergy Immunol 1999;10(1):39–44.

93. Jackson DJ, Johnston SL. The role of viruses in acute exacerbations of asthma. J Allergy Clin Immunol 2010;125(6):1178–87.

94. Stack AM, Malley R, Saladino RA, et al. Primary respiratory syncytial virus infection: pathology, immune response, and evaluation of vaccine challenge strains in a new mouse model. Vaccine 2000;18(14):1412–8.

95. Kong X, Hellermann G, Patton G, et al. An immunocompromised BALB/c mouse model for respiratory syncytial virus infection. Virology Journal 2005;2(1):3.

96. David EP, William WB, Kris AS, et al. Rhinovirus-induced PBMC responses and outcome of experimental infection in allergic subjects. J Allergy Clin Immunol 2000;105(4):692–8.

97. Nizar NJ, James EG, Elizabeth ABK, et al. The effect of an experimental rhinovirus 16 infection on bronchial lavage neutrophils. J Allergy Clin Immunol 2000; 105(6):1169–77.

98. Gern JE, Vrtis R, Grindle KA, et al. Relationship of upper and lower airway cytokines to outcome of experimental rhinovirus infection. Am J Respir Crit Care Med 2000;162(6):2226–31.

99. de Kluijver J, Gruberg K, Sont JK, et al. Rhinovirus infection in nonasthmatic subjects: effects on intrapulmonary airways. Eur Respir J 2002;20(2): 274–9.

100. DeMore JP, Weisshaar EH, Vrtis RF, et al. Similar colds in subjects with allergic asthma and nonatopic subjects after inoculation with rhinovirus-16. J Allergy Clin Immunol 2009;124(2):245–52 e3.

101. Fraenkel DJ, Bardin PG, Sanderson G, et al. Lower airways inflammation during rhinovirus colds in normal and in asthmatic subjects. Am J Respir Crit Care Med 1995;151(3):879–86.

102. Gern JE. Rhinovirus and the initiation of asthma. Curr Opin Allergy Clin Immunol 2009;9(1):73–8.

103. Wark PA, Johnston SL, Moric I, et al. Neutrophil degranulation and cell lysis is associated with clinical severity in virus-induced asthma. Eur Respir J 2002; 19(1):68–75.

104. Amin K, Ludviksdottir D, Janson C, et al. Inflammation and structural changes in the airways of patients with atopic and nonatopic asthma. Am J Respir Crit Care Med 2000;162(6):2295–301.

105. Lee FE, Walsh EE, Falsey AR, et al. Experimental infection of humans with A2 respiratory syncytial virus. Antiviral Res 2004;63(3):191–6.

106. DeVincenzo J, Lambkin-Williams R, Wilkinson T, et al. A randomized, double-blind, placebo-controlled study of an RNAi-based therapy directed against respiratory syncytial virus. Proc Natl Acad Sci 2010;107(19):8800–5.

107. Noah TL, Ivins SS, Murphy P, et al. Chemokines and inflammation in the nasal passages of infants with respiratory syncytial virus bronchiolitis. Clin Immunol 2002;104(1):86–95.

108. Noah T, Becker S. Chemokines in nasal secretions of normal adults experimentally infected with respiratory syncytial virus. Clin Immunol 2000;97(1):43–9.

109. Hornsleth A, Loland L, Larsen L. Cytokines and chemokines in respiratory secretion and severity of disease in infants with respiratory syncytial virus (RSV) infection. J Clin Virol 2001;21(2):163–70.

110. Mohapatra SS, Boyapalle S. Epidemiologic, experimental, and clinical links between respiratory syncytial virus infection and asthma. Clin Microbiol Rev 2008;21(3):495–504.

111. Olson MR, Varga SM. Pulmonary immunity and immunopathology: lessons from respiratory syncytial virus. Expert Rev Vaccines 2008;7(8):1239–55.

112. Saito T, Deskin R, Casola A, et al. Respiratory syncytial virus induces selective production of the chemokine RANTES by upper airway epithelial cells. J Infect Dis 1997;175(3):497–504.

113. Kim HH, Lee MH, Lee JS. Eosinophil cationic protein and chemokines in nasopharyngeal secretions of infants with respiratory syncytial virus (RSV) bronchiolitis and non-RSV bronchiolitis. J Korean Med Sci 2007;22(1):37–42.

114. Frigas E, Motojima S, Gleich GJ. The eosinophilic injury to the mucosa of the airways in the pathogenesis of bronchial asthma. Eur Respir J 1991;4: S123–35.

115. Venge P, Dahl R, Fredens K, et al. Epithelial injury by human eosinophils. Am Rev Respir Dis 1988;138(6):S54–7.

116. Oddera S, Silvestri M, Penna R, et al. Airway eosinophilic inflammation and bronchial hyperresponsiveness after allergen inhalation challenge in asthma. Lung 1998;176(4):237–47.

117. Kelly JT, Fox KE, Lucey EH, et al. Eosinophil regulatory activity in models of virus-induced inflammation. J Allergy Clin Immunol 2009;123(2):976.

118. Phipps S, Lam CE, Mahalingam S, et al. Eosinophils contribute to innate antiviral immunity and promote clearance of respiratory syncytial virus. Blood 2007; 110(5):1578–86.
119. Rosenberg HF, Domachowske JB. Eosinophils, eosinophil ribonucleases, and their role in host defense against respiratory virus pathogens. J Leukoc Biol 2001;70(5):691–8.
120. Davoine F, Cao M, Wu Y, et al. Virus-induced eosinophil mediator release requires antigen-presenting and CD4+ T cells. J Allergy Clin Immunol 2008; 122(1):69–77 e2.
121. Kim CK, Kim JT, Kang H, et al. Sputum eosinophilia in cough-variant asthma as a predictor of the subsequent development of classic asthma. Clin Exp Allergy 2003;33(10):1409–14.
122. Chung HL, Kim SG. RANTES may be predictive of later recurrent wheezing after respiratory syncytial virus bronchiolitis in infants. Ann Allergy Asthma Immunol 2002;88(5):463–7.
123. Pifferi M, Ragazzo V, Caramella D, et al. Eosinophil cationic protein in infants with respiratory syncytial virus bronchiolitis: predictive value for subsequent development of persistent wheezing. Pediatr Pulmonol 2001;31(6):419–24.
124. Cabalka AK. Physiologic risk factors for respiratory viral infections and immuno-prophylaxis for respiratory syncytial virus in young children with congenital heart disease. Pediatr Infect Dis J 2004;23(1):S41–5.
125. Eisenhut M. Extrapulmonary manifestations of severe respiratory syncytial virus infection—a systematic review. Crit Care 2006;10(4):6.
126. Saltzman RL, Peterson PK. Immunodeficiency of the elderly. Rev Infect Dis 1987;9(6):1127–39.
127. Schlender J, Bossert B, Buchholz U, et al. Bovine respiratory syncytial virus nonstructural proteins NS1 and NS2 cooperatively antagonize alpha/beta inter-feron-induced antiviral response. J Virol 2000;74(18):8234–42.
128. Tran KC, Collins PL, Teng MN. Effects of altering the transcription termination signals of respiratory syncytial virus on viral gene expression and growth in vitro and in vivo. J Virol 2004;78(2):692–9.
129. Gonzalez PA, Prado CE, Leiva ED, et al. Respiratory syncytial virus impairs T cell activation by preventing synapse assembly with dendritic cells. Proc Natl Acad Sci U S A 2008;105(39):14999–5004.
130. Roman M, Calhoun WJ, Hinton KL, et al. Respiratory syncytial virus infection in infants is associated with predominant Th-2-like response. Am J Respir Crit Care Med 1997;156(1):190–5.
131. Elser B, Lohoff M, Kock S, et al. IFN-gamma represses IL-4 expression via IRF-1 and IRF-2. Immunity 2002;17(6):703–12.
132. Lohoff M, Mittrucker HW, Prechtl S, et al. Dysregulated T helper cell differentia-tion in the absence of interferon regulatory factor 4. Proc Natl Acad Sci U S A 2002;99(18):11808–12.
133. Le Bon A, Tough DF. Links between innate and adaptive immunity via type I interferon. Curr Opin Immunol 2002;14(4):432–6.
134. Lohoff M, Mak TW. Roles of interferon-regulatory factors in T-helper-cell differen-tiation. Nat Rev Immunol 2005;5(2):125–35.
135. Dent AL, Hu-Li J, Paul WE, et al. T helper type 2 inflammatory disease in the absence of interleukin 4 and transcription factor STAT6. Proc Natl Acad Sci U S A 1998;95(23):13823–8.
136. Tripp RA, Jones LP, Haynes LM, et al. CX3C chemokine mimicry by respiratory syncytial virus G glycoprotein. Nat Immunol 2001;2(8):732–8.

137. Johnson TR, Graham BS. Secreted respiratory syncytial virus g glycoprotein induces Interleukin-5 (IL-5), IL-13, and eosinophilia by an IL-4-independent mechanism. J Virol 1999;73(10):8485–95.

138. Becker Y. Respiratory syncytial virus (RSV) evades the human adaptive immune system by skewing the Th1/Th2 cytokine balance toward increased levels of Th2 cytokines and IgE, markers of allergy—a review. Virus Genes 2006;33(2): 235–52.

139. Inoue D, Yamaya M, Kubo H, et al. Mechanisms of mucin production by rhinovirus infection in cultured human airway epithelial cells. Respir Physiol Neurobiol 2006;154(3):484–99.

140. Laza-Stanca V, Stanciu LA, Message SD, et al. Rhinovirus replication in human macrophages induces NF-kappa B-dependent tumor necrosis factor alpha production. J Virol 2006;80(16):8248–58.

141. Uhl EW, Clarke TJ, Hogan RJ. Differential expression of nuclear factor-kappa B mediates increased pulmonary expression of tumor necrosis factor-alpha and virus-induced asthma. Viral Immunol 2009;22(2):79–89.

142. Baldwin AS. The NF-kappa B and I kappa B proteins: new discoveries and insights. Annu Rev Immunol 1996;14:649–83.

143. Hewson CA, Jardine A, Edwards MR, et al. Toll-like receptor 3 is induced by and mediates antiviral activity against rhinovirus infection of human bronchial epithelial cells. J Virol 2005;79(19):12273–9.

144. Kurt-Jones EA, Popova L, Kwinn L, et al. Pattern recognition receptors TLR4 and CD14 mediate response to respiratory syncytial virus. Nat Immunol 2000;1(5): 398–401.

145. Monick MM, Yarovinsky TO, Powers LS, et al. Respiratory syncytial virus upregulates TLR4 and sensitizes airway epithelial cells to endotoxin. J Biol Chem 2003;278(52):53035–44.

146. Greve JM, Forte CP, Marlor CW, et al. Mechanisms of receptor-mediated rhinovirus neutralization defined by two soluble forms of ICAM-1. J Virol 1991;65(11): 6015–23.

147. Hayden FG, Gwaltney JM, Colonno RJ. Modification of experimental rhinovirus colds by receptor blockade. Antiviral Res 1988;9(4):233–47.

148. Charles CH, Luo GX, Kohlstaedt LA, et al. Prevention of human rhinovirus infection by multivalent Fab molecules directed against ICAM-1. Antimicrob Agents Chemother 2003;47(5):1503–8.

149. Fang F, Yu M. Viral receptor blockage by multivalent recombinant antibody fusion proteins: inhibiting human rhinovirus (HRV) infection with CFY196. J Antimicrob Chemother 2004;53(1):23–5.

150. Taki S, Sato T, Ogasawara K, et al. Multistage regulation of Th1-type immune responses by the transcription factor IRF-1. Immunity 1997;6(6):673–9.

151. Papadopoulos NG, Stanciu LA, Papi A, et al. A defective type 1 response to rhinovirus in atopic asthma. Thorax 2002;57(4):328–32.

152. Schwarze J, Hamelmann E, Bradley K, et al. Respiratory syncytial virus infection results in airway hyperresponsiveness and enhanced airway sensitization to allergen. J Clin Invest 1997;100(1):226–33.

153. Kotla S, Peng T, Bumgarner RE, et al. Attenuation of the type I interferon response in cells infected with human rhinovirus. Virology 2008;374(2): 399–410.

154. Rotbart HA. Treatment of picornavirus infections. Antiviral Res 2002;53(2): 83–98.

155. Kumar M, Behera A, Matsuse H, et al. Intranasal IFN-gamma gene transfer protects BALB/c mice against respiratory syncytial virus infection. Vaccine 1999;18(5-6):558–67.
156. Turner RB, Wecker MT, Pohl G, et al. Efficacy of tremacamra, a soluble intercellular adhesion molecule 1, for experimental rhinovirus infection: a randomized clinical trial. JAMA 1999;281(19):1797–804.
157. Wu H, Pfarr DS, Johnson S, et al. Development of motavizumab, an ultra-potent antibody for the prevention of respiratory syncytial virus infection in the upper and lower respiratory tract. J Mol Biol 2007;368(3):652–65.
158. Hayden FG, Herrington DT, Coats TL, et al. Efficacy and safety of oral pleconaril for treatment of colds due to picornaviruses in adults: results of 2 double-blind, randomized, placebo-controlled trials. Clin Infect Dis 2003;36(12):1523–32.
159. Meissner HC, Rennels MB, Pickering LK, et al. Risk of severe respiratory syncytial virus disease, identification of high risk infants and recommendations for prophylaxis with palivizumab. Pediatr Infect Dis J 2004;23(3):284–5.
160. The IMpact-RSV Study Group. Palivizumab, a humanized respiratory syncytial virus monoclonal antibody, reduces hospitalization from respiratory syncytial virus infection in high-risk infants. Pediatrics 1998;102(3):531–7.
161. Patick AK, Brothers MA, Maldonado F, et al. In vitro antiviral activity and single-dose pharmacokinetics in humans of a novel, orally bioavailable inhibitor of human rhinovirus 3C protease. Antimicrobial Agents Chemother 2005;49(6):2267–75.
162. Kimura K, Mori S, Tomita K, et al. Antiviral activity of NMSO3 against respiratory syncytial virus infection in vitro and in vivo. Antiviral Res 2000;47(1):41–51.
163. Stone JK, Rijnbrand R, Stein DA, et al. A morpholino oligomer targeting highly conserved internal ribosome entry site sequence is able to inhibit multiple species of picornavirus. Antimicrobial Agents Chemother 2008;52(6):1970–81.
164. Sudo K, Miyazaki Y, Kojima N, et al. YM-53403, a unique anti-respiratory syncytial virus agent with a novel mechanism of action. Antiviral Res 2005;65(2):125–31.
165. DeVincenzo J, Cehelsky JE, Alvarez R, et al. Evaluation of the safety, tolerability and pharmacokinetics of ALN-RSV01, a novel RNAi antiviral therapeutic directed against respiratory syncytial virus (RSV). Antiviral Res 2008;77(3):225–31.
166. Riccioni G, Bucciarelli T, Mancini B, et al. Antileukotriene drugs: clinical application, effectiveness and safety. Curr Med Chem 2007;14(18):1966–77.
167. Expert Panel Report 3: guidelines for the diagnosis and management of asthma. Bethesda (MD): National Heart Lung and Blood Institute; 2007.
168. Donohue JF, Ohar JA. Effects of corticosteroids on lung function in asthma and chronic obstructive pulmonary disease. Proc Am Thorac Soc 2004;1(3):152–60.
169. Panickar J, Lakhanpaul M, Lambert PC, et al. Oral prednisolone for preschool children with acute virus-induced wheezing. N Engl J Med 2009;360(4):329–38.
170. Chan MT, Leung DYM, Szefler SJ, et al. Difficult-to-control asthma: clinical characteristics of steroid-insensitive asthma. J Allergy Clin Immunol 1998;101(5):594–601.
171. Hew M, Chung KF. Corticosteroid insensitivity in severe AST HMA: significance, mechanisms and aetiology. Int Med J 2010;40(5):323–34.
172. Bisgaard H, Study Group on Montelukast and Respiratory Syncytial Virus. A randomized trial of montelukast in respiratory syncytial virus postbronchiolitis. Am J Respir Crit Care Med 2003;167(3):379–83.

173. Bisgaard H, Flores-Nunez A, Goh A, et al. Study of montelukast for the treatment of respiratory symptoms of post-respiratory syncytial virus bronchiolitis in children. Am J Respir Crit Care Med 2008;178(8):854–60.

174. Kim CK, Choi J, Kim HB, et al. A randomized intervention of montelukast for post-bronchiolitis: effect on eosinophil degranulation. J Pediatrics 2010; 156(5):749–54.

175. Friedlander SL, Jackson DJ, Gangnon RE, et al. Viral infections, cytokine dysregulation and the origins of childhood asthma and allergic diseases. Pediatr Infect Dis J 2005;24(Suppl 11):S170–6 [discussion: S174–5].

176. Simões EA, Carbonell-Estrany X, Rieger CH, et al. The effect of respiratory syncytial virus on subsequent recurrent wheezing in atopic and nonatopic children. J Allergy Clin Immunol 2010;126(2):256–62.

177. Hayden FG, Turner RB, Gwaltney JM, et al. Phase II, randomized, double-blind, placebo-controlled studies of ruprintrivir nasal spray 2-percent suspension for prevention and treatment of experimentally induced rhinovirus colds in healthy volunteers. Antimicrobial Agents Chemother 2003;47(12):3907–16.

178. Patick AK. Rhinovirus chemotherapy. Antiviral Res 2006;71(2-3):391–6.

179. Chapman J, Abbott E, Alber DG, et al. RSV604, a novel inhibitor of respiratory syncytial virus replication. Antimicrobial Agents Chemother 2007;51(9): 3346–53.

180. Cianci C, Genovesi EV, Lamb L, et al. Oral efficacy of a respiratory syncytial virus inhibitor in rodent models of infection. Antimicrobial Agents Chemother 2004;48(7):2448–54.

181. Sidwell RW, Barnard DL. Respiratory syncytial virus infections: recent prospects for control. Antiviral Res 2006;71(2–3):379–90.

182. Bitko V, Musiyenko A, Shuyayeva O, et al. Inhibition of respiratory viruses by nasally administered siRNA. Nat Med 2005;11(1):50–5.

Viral Diversity in Asthma

Peter McErlean, PhD[a],*, Alyssa Greiman, BSc[a],
Silvio Favoreto Jr, PhD, DDS[b], Pedro C. Avila, MD[c]

KEYWORDS

• Asthma • Exacerbation • Respiratory • Newly identified virus

Asthma is a heterogeneous inflammatory disease of the airways characterized by reversible airway obstruction, airway hyperresponsiveness, inflammatory cell infiltration, thickening of the lamina reticularis, and the accompanying symptoms of chest tightness, wheezing, coughing, and shortness of breath.[1,2] Asthma now affects an estimated 16.4 million adults and 7.0 million children (7.3% and 9.4% of the population, respectively) within the United States[3,4] and is additionally indicated as a "contributing factor" in nearly 7000 deaths each year.[5]

Whereas chronic asthma results from the daily inhalation and response to allergen (eg, dust, pollen, animal dander) and is by and large successfully managed by the individual, acute asthma attacks or exacerbations are precipitated primarily by respiratory viral infections and frequently require immediate medical intervention. In the United States alone, severe asthma exacerbations lead to over 400,000 hospitalizations each year, at a cost of one-third of the total $11.5 billion in annual asthma-related health care expenditures.[6]

Although the exact mechanism(s) by which respiratory viral infection causes asthma exacerbation remains to be determined, the respiratory viruses implicated in exacerbations have themselves been largely identified and well characterized (**Table 1**). Traditionally associated with acute respiratory illness (ARI) or symptoms of the "common cold," the respiratory viruses implicated in asthma exacerbations predominantly possess RNA genomes with a distinct genome organization (positive [+] or negative [−] sense), virus particle (virion) morphology (enveloped or nonenveloped), host cell receptor interaction, and well-defined annual or seasonal prevalence

Funding: Glen and Wendy Miller Family Foundation, Ernest S. Bazley Grant, NIH grant U01AI082984.
[a] Division of Allergy-Immunology, Feinberg School of Medicine, Northwestern University, 240 East Huron, McGaw M530h, Chicago, IL 60611, USA
[b] Biology Division, Cuesta College, HWY1, San Luis Obispo, CA, 93401, USA
[c] Division Allergy-Immunology, Feinberg School of Medicine, Northwestern University, 676 North Saint Claire Street, Suite 14, Chicago, IL 60611, USA
* Corresponding author.
E-mail address: p-mcerlean@northwestern.edu

Immunol Allergy Clin N Am 30 (2010) 481–495
doi:10.1016/j.iac.2010.08.001
0889-8561/10/$ – see front matter © 2010 Elsevier Inc. All rights reserved.

Table 1
Human respiratory viruses associated with asthma exacerbations

	Genome	Virion Morphology	Species or Subtypes	Cell Receptor(s)	Highest Seasonal Prevalence	% of Virus-Related Asthma Exacerbation
RNA Viruses						
Picornaviruses						
HRV (rhinovirus)	ss +ve	Nonenveloped icosahedral	A, B, C	ICAM-1, VLDL-R	Spring, Autumn	20–80
HEV[a] (enterovirus)			A–D	ICAM-1, Coxsackie-adenovirus receptor (CAR), αβ integrins	Variable	
Paramyxoviruses						
RSV (respiratory syncytial virus)	ss –ve	Enveloped pleomorphic	A, B	Heparan sulfate (HS)(?)	Late autumn–winter	5–50
HMPV (meta-pneumovirus)			(A, B?)	Integrin αvβ1	Late winter–spring	2–13
PIV (parainfluenzavirus)			1, 2, 3, 4a, 4b	Sialic acid–containing oligosaccharides	Mostly winter	1–8
Orthomyxoviruses						
IFAV (influenzavirus)	ss –ve segmented	Enveloped pleomorphic	Various	Glycans with α2,6 or α2,3 sialic acid–galactose linkages (subtype/host dependent)	Winter	1–9
IFBV						
IFCV						
Coronaviruses						
HCoV-229E	ss +ve	Enveloped pleomorphic	*Alphacoronavirus*^	CD13 (aminopeptidase N)	Autumn, winter	1–4
HCoV-NL63				Angiotensin-converting enzyme (ACE)-2	Winter, spring, summer	
HCoV-OC43			*Betacoronavirus*^	9-O-acetylated sialic acid moieties	Autumn, winter	
HCoV-HKU1				TD	Autumn, winter	

DNA Viruses

AdV (adenovirus)	ds linear	Nonenveloped icosahedral	A–F	CAR, HS-glycosaminoglycans, CD86, various integrins	Winter, spring	<7
HBoV (bocavirus)	ss circular	TD (most likely nonenveloped icosahedral)	1–3(?)	TD	Winter	6–13(?)
WuPyV (WU polyomavirus) KIPyV (KI polyomavirus)	ds circular	TD (most likely nonenveloped cosahedral)	TD	TD	Spring, autumn, winter	TD

Newly identified viruses (NIVs) are underlined.

[a] Human enteroviruses including: Coxsackieviruses and other enteroviruses associated with acute respiratory illness; ss, single-stranded; +ve, positive sense; −ve, negative sense; ds, double-stranded; (?), research ongoing; ^, genera of the subfamily *Coronavirinae*; TD, to be determined.

The full extent of respiratory virus involvement in exacerbation has recently been revealed in asthma studies with the implementation of molecular methods of viral detection, specifically the reverse transcriptase polymerase chain reaction (RT-PCR).[7,8] Molecular methods of viral detection have superior sensitivity and specificity compared with cell culture–based methods and additionally allow for the improved identification of multiple viruses (and other pathogens), revealing the role dual or multiple infections play in asthma exacerbations. Indeed, molecular methods have also been invaluable in identifying new respiratory viruses, the majority of which were described after the emergence of the severe acute respiratory syndrome-associated coronavirus (SARS-CoV) that prompted research into the etiology of ARI. These "newly identified viruses" (NIVs) including human metapneumovirus (HMPV; described pre-SARS), the human rhinovirus (HRV) species C (HRV-Cs), human coronaviruses (HCoVs)-NL63 and -HKU1, human bocavirus (HBoV), and the KI and WU polyomaviruses (KIPyV and WUPyV) are now the focus of intense research, and their involvement in asthma exacerbations is slowly beginning to be determined.

Because those respiratory viruses most associated with exacerbations—the HRVs, respiratory syncytial virus (RSV), and HMPV—are reviewed elsewhere in this issue by Miller and colleagues, this review discusses some of the other respiratory viruses implicated in childhood and adult asthma exacerbations, including additional RNA viruses and those with DNA genomes. By also encompassing some of the recently described NIVs, this article illustrates the diversity that exists in virus-related asthma exacerbations.

INFLUENZA VIRUSES

Influenza viruses (IFVs) are probably the best known of all the respiratory viruses, due to their ability to cause annual epidemics and potential pandemics of serious respiratory disease.[9] IFVs pose the greatest risk of morbidity and mortality to young children and the elderly, and as such have been the focus of repeated public health and vaccination campaigns. However, despite their potential to cause serious respiratory illness in otherwise healthy individuals, most asthma studies describe relatively low levels of IFVs in exacerbations, accounting for approximately 1% to 9% of all virus-related asthma exacerbations (see **Table 1**).[7,10–16]

IFVs constitute the family *Orthomyxoviridae* and are segmented −single stranded (ss) RNA viruses. The IFV virion has a pleomorphic envelope derived from host cell membranes and incorporates 3 viral encoded surface proteins: hemagglutinin (HA), neuraminidase (NA), and matrix protein 2 (M2). Under the envelope and encased within the matrix protein (M1), the core of the IFV virion contains the ribonucleoprotein complex, consisting of the viral RNA segments, polymerase proteins (PB1, PB2, and PA), and the nucleoprotein (NP).[17]

There are 3 types of IFVs, -A (IFAV), -B (IFBV), and -C (IFCV), which are divided further in subtypes and strains based on the combination of HA and NA proteins (eg, H1N1, H3N2). IFAV and IFCV have subtypes known to infect both animals (eg, birds, pigs) and humans, whereas IFBV is predominately a human virus. Although all types of IFVs can cause ARI in humans, IFAV and IFBV subtypes and strains are of the most prominent in the annual epidemics or "flu season" that occurs during the winter months.

IFVs initiate infection via the HA protein attaching to sialic acid (SA) linked to galactose (Gal) sugars on the terminal ends of host cell surface glycans. It has been determined that the HA interaction is dependent on the sialic acid-galactose linkages, with HA from subtypes that infect humans recognizing $\alpha2,6$ linkages (SAα2,6Gal), whereas

HA from subtypes infecting other animals mostly recognize $\alpha2,3$ linkages (SAα2,3Gal).[17,18]

Although IFVs are implicated in 1.9% to 6.6% of wheezing illnesses in children[7,10,12,13] and have been detected in 9.8% of asthmatic adults during emergency department (ED) visits,[15] uncertainty remains as to whether IFVs are specifically responsible for the production of asthma exacerbations.[19,20] The main contention arises from the role that vaccination has played in preventing exacerbations. Because, unlike other respiratory viruses, vaccines against IFV subtypes and strains are available and asthmatics frequently have increased vaccination rates due to their at-risk status during flu season, IFV-related exacerbations should be reduced or indeed eliminated among asthmatic children and adults.[21,22] However, some studies have shown that despite their three- to fourfold greater odds of having an influenza vaccination (as reported by parents), asthmatic children have higher rates of IFV-related hospital visits[23] and that vaccination does not affect the number, duration, or severity of IFV-related asthma exacerbations compared with placebo.[24] Other similar studies have shown that influenza vaccination also fails to reduce severe and fatal complications in adults with asthma and chronic obstructive pulmonary disease (COPD).[20]

The association of IFVs with exacerbations in vaccinated asthmatics questions the efficacy of seasonal influenza vaccines in this group and also suggests a role for other respiratory viruses in IFV-related exacerbations. If influenza vaccinations are effective, then it is likely that IFV-related exacerbations are caused by infection with another respiratory virus, such as those that peak in prevalence during the same time as IFVs (eg, RSV and HMPV). However, if influenza vaccination of asthmatics fails to reduce IFV-*proven* exacerbations (ie, by RT-PCR during symptomatic illness) then alternative vaccination strategies may be required to increase efficacy. Ensuring that comprehensive respiratory virus testing is employed during both influenza vaccination and asthma studies and that vaccination rates among asthmatics remain high, the contention over vaccination and IFV-related exacerbations will be better clarified.

Some recent studies focusing on ARI suggest that infection with other respiratory viruses, particularly HRVs, may actually provide "protection" against IFV infection.[25,26] Although such claims remain to be fully substantiated, viral competition may be a contributing factor in the relatively low rates of IFV-related asthma exacerbations being reported. It remains to be determined whether the asthmatic phenotype preferentially facilitates infection with respiratory viruses other than IFVs or whether, owing to vaccination in the wider community, the overall prevalence of IFVs is reduced making infection with another "uncontrolled" respiratory virus more likely.

The association of IFVs with asthma exacerbation is complicated by the emergence of more virulent pandemic strains, such as the novel 2009 swine-origin IFAV H1N1 (S-OIV), which may pose a greater risk to asthmatics than seasonal strains.[27] Although the full impact of S-OIV remains to be determined, initial studies have indicated that among both children and adults hospitalized with RT-PCR–identified S-OIV, asthma accounted for the largest percentage (28%) of all underlying medical conditions.[27] However, it is unclear whether S-OIV evokes a specific immune response among asthmatics or whether, owing to increased awareness of this particular strain, asthmatics were more likely to seek medical care when respiratory symptoms initially began.

HUMAN CORONAVIRUSES

HCoVs were initially described in the 1960s in studies aiming to determine the etiologic agent responsible for ARI, but gained notoriety after the emergence of SARS-CoV in 2003. Since that time, 2 additional HCoVs have been described in ARI studies, indicating that there are several HCoVs potentially associated with respiratory illness in humans. Because of the severity of associated illness, this review excludes SARS-CoV and focuses solely on the 4 HCoVs associated with ARI and currently implicated in 1% to 4% of virus-related asthma exacerbations: HCoV-OC43, HCoV-229E, and the NIVs, HCoV-NL63 and HCoV-HKU1 (see **Table 1**).[10,12,28,29]

HCoVs are classified within the Family *Coronaviridae*, subfamily *Coronavirinae*, with the Genus *Alphacoronavirus* containing HCoV-229E and HCoV-NL63 and the Genus *Betacoronavirus* containing HCoV-OC43 and HCoV-HKU1.[30] HCoVs possess a +ssRNA genome, which is associated with nucleocapsid (N) phosphoprotein within the core of a host cell–derived enveloped virion. The HCoV virion also comprises 3 viral encoded proteins (S, E, and M), and characterization has indicated that binding to host cell receptors is mediated predominately via the spike (S) glycoprotein, with each HCoV employing a specific host cell receptor during infection (see **Table 1**). The virion of *Betacoronavirus* also contains a hemagglutinin (HE) protein, which is thought to be involved in either host-receptor interactions or release of virus from infected cells.[31–33]

The molecular and receptor interaction differences existing between HCoVs are reflected in their seasonal prevalences. Studies of ARI have indicated that HCoV-NL63 can be detected in the spring, summer, or winter whereas HCoVs -HKU1, -OC43, and -229E infections mainly occur during the autumn and winter months.[34–37] A recent study of HCoVs -NL63, -OC43, and -229E also found fluctuations occurring between their yearly prevalence.[37]

The clinical impact of each HCoV also appears to vary, but all present the greatest disease burden within the childhood population.[34] In a retrospective study of clinical samples taken over a 20-year period from young children (median age 14.5 months), the percentage of lower respiratory tract illness (LRTI; including asthma exacerbations and bronchiolitis) associated with any HCoV, HCoV-NL63, or HCoV-OC43 was estimated to be 4.6%, 2.6%, and 1.9%, respectively.[37] Although this study failed to include HCoV-HKU1 in the testing panels, other studies have associated HCoV-HKU1 with wheezing illness in children.[34,38]

Among asthmatic adults, HCoVs have been detected during both ED visits and well-defined episodes of exacerbation prompted by ARI. Atmar and colleagues[15] reported that HCoVs were detected in 21 of 148 ED visits during a 2-year study of 122 asthmatic adults, and Kistler and colleagues[39] reported detections of HCoVs, OC43, HKU1, and NL63 in asthmatic adults with ARI, of which HCoV-NL63 occurred most in episodes of exacerbations.

Despite being associated with ARI, HCoV-229E appears to be the HCoV least associated with asthma exacerbations. Recent studies using RT-PCR have failed to find HCoV-229E in either adult or childhood episodes of asthma exacerbation.[34,37,39] Although some previous studies detected HCoV-229E in asthmatic children, detection occurred with HCoV-OC43 and individual HCoV detection rates were not reported, despite the investigators using HCoV-OC43- and HCoV-229E–specific primers and antibodies.[16] Another early study of asthmatic adults detected HCoV-229E through analysis of paired sera in 12 instances where exacerbation could be objectively measured. However, HCoV-299E detections could not be associated with a peak expiratory flow rate (PEFR) mean decrease of greater than 50 L/min.[40] The reason for the lack of HCoV-229E detections in asthma exacerbations remains unclear.

PARAINFLUENZA VIRUSES

Parainfluenza viruses (PIVs) are primarily associated with bronchiolitis and laryngotracheobronchitis or croup, in children younger than 4 years of age.[41,42] PIVs also pose a serious risk to immunocompromised individuals, and outbreaks of viral pneumonia among transplant recipients and patients undergoing chemotherapy have occurred.[41,42] The PIVs consist of 4 serotypes (1–4) and 2 subtypes (4a and 4b), and as a group are responsible for 1% to 8% of virus-related asthma exacerbations (see **Table 1**).[7,10,12,13,29,43]

Like RSV and HMPV, PIVs are nonsegmented −ssRNA viruses belonging to the family *Paramyxoviridae*.[44] PIVs 1 to 3, 4a, and 4b are classified within 2 of the 5 genera of the subfamily *Paramyxovirinae,* genus Respirovirus (PIV-1 and PIV-3) and genus *Rubulavirus* (PIV2 and PIV 4a and -4b).[45] In contrast to the G glycoprotein encoded by RSV and HMPV, PIVs encode a hemagglutinin-neuraminidase (HN) glycoprotein, which interacts with gangliosides (sialic acid–containing oligosaccharides) on target host cells during infection.[46,47]

Seasonal and yearly prevalence of PIVs have been shown to vary among the serotypes. PIV-1, -2, and -4 have the highest prevalence in the autumn and winter months whereas PIV-3 occurs mostly in the spring and summer. Peaks in PIV-1 prevalence have been shown to occur biennially. PIV-2 prevalence exhibits some yearly variation and PIV-3 is consistently detected each year. PIV-4 is the least prevalent of all PIVs.[42] Although each PIV has the potential to cause respiratory illness in any age group, PIVs 1 to 3 appear to be more associated with a particular clinical presentation at certain ages. PIV-1 is associated with croup in children 1 to 4 years old, PIV-2 with bronchiolitis in the age group younger than 1 year, and PIV-3 is more associated with viral pneumonia in individuals older than 15 years.[42]

Studies of asthmatic children have revealed that each PIV type plays a different role in the production of asthma symptoms. In studies where the incidence of each individual PIV is described, PIV-1 is detected in 1.4% to 2.9%, PIV-2 in 1.4%, PIV-3 in 2.9% to 6%, and PIV-4 in up to 1.9% of wheezing illnesses.[12–14,43] Although PIVs are largely considered as a single group in adult asthma studies, PIVs are still detected in episodes of exacerbation. Atmar and colleagues[15] detected PIVs 1 to 3 in 16 of 138 episodes of ARI in asthmatic adults, with at least one infection each of PIV-2 and PIV-3 resulting in an ED visit, and Nicholson and colleagues[40] detected 5 cases of PIV1-3 in asthmatic adults, 3 of which had instances of a PEFR mean decrease of greater than 50 L/min.

ADENOVIRUSES

Adenoviruses (AdVs) comprise a large group of DNA viruses that are known to cause a wide variety of clinical syndromes including diarrhea, keratoconjunctivitis, and hemorrhagic cystitis.[48,49] However, AdVs are best known as a primary cause of ARI and, particularly in young children, have been implicated in the production of more severe LRTI. Fifty-one AdV serotypes have been identified, and as a group AdVs are associated with up to 7% of virus-related asthma exacerbations (see **Table 1**).[7,10,13,29,43]

AdVs are classified within the family *Adenoviridae*, genus *Mastadenovirus*, and divided into species A through G based on biochemical and biophysical properties, hemagglutination reaction, and sequence identity. The AdV virion is a nonenveloped icosahedral capsid consisting of 240 hexon and 12 penton polyproteins or capsomers. A long fiber protein protrudes from each of the 12 penton capsomers and contains a terminal "knob" domain, which interacts with host cell receptors.[49] AdVs have been shown to employ a diverse variety of cell receptors, including coxsackie-adenovirus receptor (CAR), heparan sulfate glycosaminoglycans, CD86, and an array of cell surface integrins.[50]

Although each serotype exhibits some variation, AdVs are detected primarily during the winter and spring months.[10,48] Of all the serotypes, AdV-1, -2, -5, and -6 are the most common cause of ARI.[51,52] However, similar to other respiratory viruses (eg, RSV subtype detections reported by Lee and colleagues[12] versus Matthew and colleagues[14]), location can affect the predominance of a given serotype, with AdV-4, -7, and -5 being the most frequently detected in ARI studies conducted in the United States.[52,53]

As with most respiratory viruses, AdV infections occur primarily in infants and children, and it is within these populations specifically that AdVs have been associated with more serious respiratory illness.[48,52,54–56] In an 8-year study of children younger than 2 years hospitalized with LRTI, Larranaga and colleagues[55] detected AdV at a rate of 8.6% (sole detections), second only to RSV (26.3%), and predominately in patients with pneumonia and wheezing bronchitis (69.8%). The investigators also typed the AdV isolates and determined that the species B and C were most frequently detected among their population and that serotype-7h was particularly associated with a longer duration of hospitalization. Although this study employed culture-based methods of detection, more recent studies employing PCR for AdV detection describe comparable detection rates (0.4%–7%) in episodes of childhood wheeze and asthma exacerbations.[7,10,13,29,43]

An interesting aspect of the association of AdV with asthma was described in a study of asymptomatic asthmatic children conducted by Marin and colleagues.[56] These investigators reported that AdV DNA was detected in 78.4% of the asthmatic group but in only 5% of the nonasthmatic control group. This study also described HRV and RSV detection rates in the asthmatic group of 32.4% and 2.7%, respectively, despite none of the participants experiencing respiratory symptoms for the duration of the study (3 weeks). However, a confounding aspect of this study is that the subjects were classified as having mild asthma that was well controlled (fluticasone 100–250 µg daily) in the 6 months before the start of the study. Nevertheless, the disparity in viral detection between the asthmatic and control groups may imply some mechanism of either persistence in asthmatics or an association with the long-term compliance of glucocorticoid therapy and inhibition of symptoms during respiratory virus infection.

HUMAN BOCAVIRUSES

Human bocaviruses (HBoV) were discovered in 2005 by Allander and colleagues[57] in pooled nasopharyngeal aspirates obtained from children with LRTI. Further characterization in ARI-focused studies has revealed that HBoV is frequently associated with ARI in both children and adults, with detection rates of 1.5% to 19%.[58–61] In addition, HBoV has been associated with wheezing and gastrointestinal illness predominately in children younger than 2 years.[57,61–75] However, the exact role of HBoV in respiratory and other illnesses remains ambiguous, with a high overall codetection rate with other respiratory viruses being described (median 42.5%) and the detection of HBoV DNA in serum, urine, and lymph node samples.[60,61,66,76,77]

HBoV is a parvovirus, a single-stranded DNA virus of the family *Parvoviridae,* genus *Bocavirus.*[65] The genome, which requires host cell DNA polymerases for replication, encodes 2 structural (VP1 and VP2) and 2 nonstructural (NS1 and NP1) proteins.[65] Although HBoV has only recently been propagated in cultured cells and its host cell interactions remain to be determined,[78] initial studies have found that HBoV shares similar virion morphology with other parvoviruses, a nonenveloped icosahedral capsid consisting of 60 copies of each structural protein.[79] Recently, 2 viruses related to HBoV have been identified, namely HBoV-2 and HBoV-3, but it is unknown whether these are unique viral entities or closely related genotypes of the same virus.[80,81] While the epidemiology of HBoV is still being determined, ARI studies have shown that HBoV infection occurs primarily during the winter, with a smaller peak in spring.[65,74,82]

Several studies have indicated that HBoV is associated with severe respiratory disease in children, particularly in those hospitalized with asthma and other wheezing illnesses.[29,65] A study conducted by Vallet and colleagues[83] of children aged 2 to 15 years hospitalized for asthma detected HBoV in 13% of children with asthma exacerbations compared with only 2% in children with stable asthma, suggesting HBoV plays a causative role in the development of exacerbations. Similar findings were reported by Nadji and colleagues,[84] who detected HBoV at a rate of 6% in children younger than 10 years with asthma exacerbations, and Garcia and colleagues,[69] who reported that wheezing was seen in more than 50% of children in whom HBoV was the sole virus detected.

Although HBoV is more often detected in symptomatic than healthy individuals, high levels of codetection with other respiratory viruses, particularly picornaviruses and IFVs, confounds HBoV's role in respiratory illness.[25,65] Although a study of infants younger than 12 months hospitalized with bronchiolitis found that dual infections of RSV and HBoV were associated with higher clinical severity scores and longer length of hospitalization than infants with a single HBoV or HRV and HBoV dual infections,[85] most studies have found that coinfection of HBoV with another respiratory virus does not alter the severity or duration of associated illness.

POLYOMAVIRUSES

In 2007, 2 novel human polyomaviruses (PyVs) were described, the KI polyomavirus (KIPyV) by Allander and colleagues[86] and the WU polyomavirus (WUPyV) by Gaynor and colleagues.[87] Initially identified in nasopharyngeal aspirates obtained from individuals with respiratory illness, further characterization has revealed KIPyV and WUPyV are detected in 2.6% and 6.2% of ARI cases, respectively, suggesting these NIVs have a causative role in respiratory illnesses.[88-91] However, similar to HBoV, a high rate of codetection (>80%) with other respiratory viruses and detection in other tissue types currently confounds any direct association of KIPyV and WUPyV with ARI and other illnesses.[92]

PyVs are classified in the single genus *Polyomavirus* of the family *Polyomaviridae*, and contain histone-associated circular dsDNA genomes encoding 3 structural (VP1, VP2, VP3) and 2 nonstructural (large-T and small-T antigens) proteins.[87,93] As with some other NIVs (eg, HRV C, HCoV-HKU1), KIPyV and WUPyV cannot be grown using current cell culture systems. This drawback has postponed identification of host cell receptor interactions and determination of virion morphology, although the latter is believed to be similar to the nonenveloped icosahedral configuration of other PyVs.[93]

KIPyV and WUPyV characterization in retrospective ARI-focused studies has determined that they exhibit a year-round prevalence, with the greatest peaks in detections occurring in the spring, autumn, and winter months.[90,94-96] Although no studies have yet looked specifically for KIPyV and WUPyV during episodes of asthma exacerbations, wheezing illness and other more serious LRTI have been reported in patients positive for KIPyV and WUPyV. Bialasiewicz and colleagues[90] showed that 15% of KIPyV-positive and 23% of WUPyV-positive patients had symptoms of bronchiolitis, and Payungporn and colleagues[96] found that 11 of 15 combined KIPyV and WUPyV sole detections originated in children younger than 1 year with pneumonia. However, the overall high codetection rates (35%–80%) described in these studies again indicates the need for further clarification of the role of KIPyV and WUPyV in respiratory illness.

An interesting aspect of the previously described human PyVs is their ability to establish a form of latency (ie, low-level persistent infection) and undergo reactivation when an infected individual's immune system experiences stress (eg, infection, inflammation, or immune suppression).[93,97] While characterization of the host-virus interactions of KIPyV and WUPyV is still continuing, Sharp and colleagues[98] have proposed that they may also reactivate during illness, as evidenced by mutations in the transcriptional control region of KIPyV and WUPyV genomes detected in autopsy tissue from immunosuppressed individuals. Given our incomplete knowledge about the role of KIPyV and WUPyV in respiratory illness, it may be plausible that the high codetection rates observed in ARI studies are not the result of bona fide dual infections, but rather may be caused by infection with another respiratory virus evoking an immune response that reactivates latent KIPyV and WUPyV.

Although Sharp and colleagues[98] did not observe the high frequency of transcriptional control region mutations in KIPyV and WUPyV genomes detected from respiratory samples, a seroepidemiology study by Nguyen and colleagues[99] may provide evidence of KIPyV and WUPyV reactivation during ARI. These investigators observed that the proportion of KIPyV- and WUPyV-seropositive individuals increased at around 4 years of age, a finding that they speculated was the result of KIPyV and WUPyV exposure during school attendance. However, they conceded that the serum obtained for their study originated from 2 tertiary referral hospitals and was likely from individuals with underlying medical conditions. Given that ARI represents the most common reason for hospital visits and admissions among school-aged children, and that the incidence of other respiratory virus infections also increases among this age group, the KIPyV and WUPyV antibody detected may not be that produced in response to initial exposure, but rather antibody produced during KIPyV and WUPyV reactivation evoked by infection with another ARI-causing respiratory virus. Indeed, Nguyen and colleagues[99] reported that a high proportion of adults were KIPyV- and WUPyV-seropositive which, considering the nature of the study cohort (ie, hospital-based), may not indicate preexisting immunity but again KIPyV and WUPyV reactivation during illness. Future community-based studies will no doubt determine when initial KIPyV and WUPyV exposure occurs and will better elucidate the relationships that exist between ARI, viral codetections, and KIPyV and WUPyV reactivation.

SUMMARY

This review focuses on some of the less common respiratory viruses currently implicated in both childhood and adult asthma exacerbations. Although the respiratory viruses covered here have a lesser, or in the case of NIVs, an as yet uncharacterized involvement in the development of exacerbation compared with the "usual suspects" (eg, HRV, RSV, HMPV), they exemplify the diversity that exists in virus-related exacerbations. The implementation of more sensitive methods of virus detection and the identification and characterization of NIVs in future asthma studies will further expand our understanding of viral diversity and the mechanisms underlying development of asthma exacerbations during respiratory virus infection.

REFERENCES

1. Grunberg K, Timmers MC, de Klerk EP, et al. Experimental rhinovirus 16 infection causes variable airway obstruction in subjects with atopic asthma. Am J Respir Crit Care Med 1999;160(4):1375–80.
2. Akinbami L. The state of childhood asthma, United States, 1980-2005. Adv Data 2006;381:1–24.

3. Pleis JRLJ, Ward BW. Summary health statistics for U.S. adults: National Health Interview Survey, 2008. National Center for Health Statistics. Vital Health Stat 2009;10:16 20–2.

4. Trends in asthma morbidity and mortality. Available at: http://www.lungusa.org/finding-cures/for-professionals/asthma-trend-report.pdf. 2010. Accessed March 2, 2010.

5. Krishnan V, Diette GB, Rand CS, et al. Mortality in patients hospitalized for asthma exacerbations in the United States. Am J Respir Crit Care Med 2006;174(6): 633–8.

6. Barnes PJ, Godfrey S. Asthma. 2nd edition. London: Informa Healthcare; 2000.

7. Jartti T, Lehtinen P, Vuorinen T, et al. Respiratory picornaviruses and respiratory syncytial virus as causative agents of acute expiratory wheezing in children. Emerg Infect Dis 2004;10(6):1095–101.

8. Jartti T, Waris M, Niesters HG, et al. Respiratory viruses and acute asthma in children. J Allergy Clin Immunol 2007;120(1):216 author reply 217.

9. Wright PF, Neumann G, Kawaoka Y. Orthomyxoviruses. In: Knipe DM, Howley PM, editors. 5th edition. Fields virology, vol. 2. Philadelphia: Lippincott-Raven; 2005. p. 1692–740.

10. Cheuk DK, Tang IW, Chan KH, et al. Rhinovirus infection in hospitalized children in Hong Kong: a prospective study. Pediatr Infect Dis J 2007;26(11):995–1000.

11. Williams JF, Crowe JE, Enriquez R, et al. Human metapneumovirus infection plays an etiologic role in acute asthma exacerbations requiring hospitalization in adults. J Infect Dis 2005;192:1149–53.

12. Lee WM, Grindle K, Pappas T, et al. High-throughput, sensitive, and accurate multiplex PCR-microsphere flow cytometry system for large-scale comprehensive detection of respiratory viruses. J Clin Microbiol 2007;45(8):2626–34.

13. Rawlinson WD, Waliuzzaman Z, Carter IW, et al. Asthma exacerbations in children are associated with rhinovirus but not human metapneumovirus infection. J Infect Dis 2003;187:1314–8.

14. Matthew J, Pinto Pereira LM, Pappas TE, et al. Distribution and seasonality of rhinovirus and other respiratory viruses in a cross-section of asthmatic children in Trinidad, West Indies. Ital J Pediatr 2009;35:16.

15. Atmar RL, Guy E, Guntupalli KK, et al. Respiratory tract viral infections in inner-city asthmatic adults. Arch Intern Med 1998;158(22):2453–9.

16. Johnston SL, Pattemore PK, Sanderson G, et al. Community study of role of viral infections in exacerbations of asthma in 9-11 year old children. BMJ 1995; 310(6989):1225–9.

17. Palese P, Shaw ML. *Orthomyxoviridae*: the viruses and their replication. In: Knipe DM, Howley PM, editors, Fields virology, vol. 2. Philadelphia: Lippincott-Raven; 2005. p. 1647–89.

18. Suzuki Y, Ito T, Suzuki T, et al. Sialic acid species as a determinant of the host range of Influenza A viruses. J Virol 2000;74(24):11825–31.

19. Jartti T, Ruuskanen O. Influenza virus and acute asthma in children. Pediatrics 2008;121(5):1079–80.

20. Bueving HJ, Thomas S, Wouden JC. Is influenza vaccination in asthma helpful? Curr Opin Allergy Clin Immunol 2005;5(1):65–70.

21. Daley MF, Barrow J, Pearson K, et al. Identification and recall of children with chronic medical conditions for influenza vaccination. Pediatrics 2004;113(1): e26–33.

22. Ford ES, Mannino DM, Williams SG. Asthma and influenza vaccination. Chest 2003;124(3):783–9.

23. Miller EK, Griffin MR, Edwards KM, et al. Influenza burden for children with asthma. Pediatrics 2008;121(1):1–8.

24. Bueving HJ, Bernsen RMD, de Jongste JC, et al. Influenza vaccination in children with asthma: randomized double-blind placebo-controlled trial. Am J Respir Crit Care Med 2004;169(4):488–93.

25. Greer RM, McErlean P, Arden KE, et al. Do rhinoviruses reduce the probability of viral co-detection during acute respiratory tract infections? J Clin Virol 2009;45(1):10–5.

26. Casalegno JS, Ottmann M, Duchamp MB, et al. Rhinoviruses delayed the circulation of the pandemic influenza A (H1N1) 2009 virus in France. Clin Microbiol Infect 2010;16(4):326–9.

27. Jain S, Kamimoto L, Bramley AM, et al. Hospitalized Patients with 2009 H1N1 Influenza in the United States, April-June 2009. N Engl J Med 2009;361(20): 1935–44.

28. Smuts H, Workman L, Zar HJ. Role of human metapneumovirus, human coronavirus NL63 and human bocavirus in infants and young children with acute wheezing. J Med Virol 2008;80(5):906–12.

29. Allander T, Jartti T, Gupta S, et al. Human bocavirus and acute wheezing in children. Clin Infect Dis 2007;44(7):904–10.

30. Virus Taxonomy: 2009 release. International Committee on Taxonomy of Viruses. Available at: http://www.ictvonline.org/virusTaxonomy.asp?version=2009. 2009. Accessed June 6, 2010.

31. Hofmann H, Pyrc K, van der Hoek L, et al. Human coronavirus NL63 employs the severe acute respiratory syndrome coronavirus receptor for cellular entry. Proc Natl Acad Sci U S A 2005;102(22):7988–93.

32. Yeager CL, Ashmun RA, Williams RK, et al. Human aminopeptidase N is a receptor for human coronavirus 229E. Nature 1992;357(6377):420–2.

33. Lai MMC, Perlman S, Anderson LJ. *Coronaviridae*: the viruses and their replication. In: Knipe PM, Howley PM, editors, Fields virology, vol. 1. Philadelphia: Lippincott-Raven; 2005. p. 1305–35.

34. Lau SKP, Woo PCY, Yip CCY, et al. Coronavirus HKU1 and other coronavirus infections in Hong Kong. J Clin Microbiol 2006;44(6):2063–71.

35. El-Sahly Hana M, Atmar Robert L, Glezen William P, et al. Spectrum of clinical illness in hospitalized patients with "common cold" virus infections. Clin Infect Dis 2000;31(1):96–100.

36. Chiu SS, Chan KH, Chu KW, et al. Human coronavirus NL63 infection and other coronavirus infections in children hospitalized with acute respiratory disease in Hong Kong, China. Clin Infect Dis 2005;40:1721–9.

37. Talbot HK, Shepherd BE, Crowe JEJ, et al. The pediatric burden of human coronaviruses evaluated for twenty years. Pediatr Infect Dis J 2009;28(8):682–7.

38. Sloots TP, McErlean P, Speicher DJ, et al. Evidence of human coronavirus HKU1 and human bocavirus in Australian children. J Clin Virol 2006;35(1):99–102.

39. Kistler A, Avila PC, Rouskin S, et al. Pan-viral screening of respiratory tract infections in adults with and without asthma reveals unexpected human coronavirus and human rhinovirus diversity. J Infect Dis 2007;196(6):817–25.

40. Nicholson KG, Kent J, Ireland DC. Respiratory viruses and exacerbations of asthma in adults. BMJ 1993;307(6910):982–6.

41. Hall CB. Respiratory syncytial virus and parainfluenza virus. N Engl J Med 2001; 344(25):1917–28.

42. Laurichesse H, Dedman D, Watson JM, et al. Epidemiological features of parainfluenza virus infections: Laboratory surveillance in England and Wales, 1975-1997. Eur J Epidemiol 1999;15(5):475–84.

43. Ong BH, Gao Q, Phoon MC, et al. Identification of human metapneumovirus and *Chlamydophila pneumoniae* in children with asthma and wheeze in Singapore. Singapore Med J 2007;48(4):291–3.
44. Lamb RA, Parks GD. Paramyxoviridae: the viruses and their replication. In: Knipe DM, Howley PM, editors, Fields virology, vol. 1. Philadelphia: Lippincott-Raven; 2005. p. 1450–96.
45. Karron RA, Collins PA. Parainfluenza viruses. In: Knipe DM, Howley PM, editors. Fields virology. Philadelphia: Lippincott-Raven; 2005. p. 1497–527.
46. Villar E, Barroso I. Role of sialic acid-containing molecules in paramyxovirus entry into the host cell: a minireview. Glycoconj J 2006;23(1):5–17.
47. Suzuki T, Portner A, Scroggs RA, et al. Receptor specificities of human respiroviruses. J Virol 2001;75(10):4604–13.
48. Brodzinski H, Ruddy RM. Review of new and newly discovered respiratory tract viruses in children. Pediatr Emerg Care 2009;25(5):352–60 quiz 361–353.
49. Berk AJ. *Adenoviridae*: the viruses and their replication. In: Knipe DM, Howley PM, editors, Fields virology, vol. 2. Philadelphia: Lippincott-Raven; 2005. p. 2355–94.
50. Zhang Y, Bergelson JM. Adenovirus receptors. J Virol 2005;79(19):12125–31.
51. Horwitz M. Adenoviruses. 3rd edition. Philadelphia: Lippincott-Raven; 1995.
52. Moro MR, Bonville CA, Suryadevara M, et al. Clinical features, adenovirus types, and local production of inflammatory mediators in adenovirus infections. Pediatr Infect Dis J 2009;28(5):376–80.
53. Foy H. Adenoviruses. 4th edition. New York: Plenum; 1997.
54. Chen HL, Chiou SS, Hsiao HP, et al. Respiratory adenoviral infections in children: a study of hospitalized cases in southern Taiwan in 2001–2002. J Trop Pediatr 2004;50(5):279–84.
55. Larranaga C, Kajon A, Villagra E, et al. Adenovirus surveillance on children hospitalized for acute lower respiratory infections in Chile (1988–1996). J Med Virol 2000;60(3):342–6.
56. Marin J, Jeler-Kacar D, Levstek V, et al. Persistence of viruses in upper respiratory tract of children with asthma. J Infect 2000;41(1):69–72.
57. Allander T, Tammi MT, Eriksson M, et al. Cloning of a human parvovirus by molecular screening of respiratory tract samples. Proc Natl Acad Sci U S A 2005; 102(36):12891–6.
58. Allander T. Human bocavirus. J Clin Virol 2008;41(1):29–33.
59. Lindner J, Karalar L, Schimanski S, et al. Clinical and epidemiological aspects of human bocavirus infection. J Clin Virol 2008;43(4):391–5.
60. Tozer SJ, Lambert SB, Whiley DM, et al. Detection of human bocavirus in respiratory, fecal, and blood samples by real-time PCR. J Med Virol 2009;81(3): 488–93.
61. Wang K, Wang W, Yan H, et al. Correlation between bocavirus infection and humoral response, and co-infection with other respiratory viruses in children with acute respiratory infection. J Clin Virol 2010;47(2):148–55.
62. Arnold JC, Singh KK, Spector SA, et al. Human bocavirus: prevalence and clinical spectrum at a children's hospital. Clin Infect Dis 2006;43(3):283–8.
63. Bastien N, Brandt K, Dust K, et al. Human bocavirus infection, Canada. Emerg Infect Dis 2006;12(5):848–50.
64. Canducci F, Debiaggi M, Sampaolo M, et al. Two-year prospective study of single infections and co-infections by respiratory syncytial virus and viruses identified recently in infants with acute respiratory disease. J Med Virol 2008;80(4):716–23.

65. Chow BD, Esper FP. The human bocaviruses: a review and discussion of their role in infection. Clin Lab Med 2009;29(4):695–713.
66. Chow BD, Huang YT, Esper FP. Evidence of human bocavirus circulating in children and adults, Cleveland, Ohio. J Clin Virol 2008;43(3):302–6.
67. Chung JY, Han TH, Kim CK, et al. Bocavirus infection in hospitalized children, South Korea. Emerg Infect Dis 2006;12(8):1254–6.
68. Fry AM, Lu X, Chittaganpitch M, et al. Human bocavirus: a novel parvovirus epidemiologically associated with pneumonia requiring hospitalization in Thailand. J Infect Dis 2007;195(7):1038–45.
69. Calvo C, Garcia-Garcia ML, Pozo F, et al. Clinical characteristics of human bocavirus infections compared with other respiratory viruses in Spanish children. Pediatr Infect Dis J 2008;27(8):677–80.
70. Garcia-Garcia ML, Calvo C, Pozo F, et al. Human bocavirus detection in nasopharyngeal aspirates of children without clinical symptoms of respiratory infection. Pediatr Infect Dis J 2008;27(4):358–60.
71. Kesebir D, Vazquez M, Weibel C, et al. Human bocavirus infection in young children in the United States: molecular epidemiological profile and clinical characteristics of a newly emerging respiratory virus. J Infect Dis 2006; 194(9):1276–82.
72. Maggi F, Andreoli E, Pifferi M, et al. Human bocavirus in Italian patients with respiratory diseases. J Clin Virol 2007;38(4):321–5.
73. Manning A, Russell V, Eastick K, et al. Epidemiological profile and clinical associations of human bocavirus and other human parvoviruses. J Infect Dis 2006; 194(9):1283–90.
74. Miron D, Srugo I, Kra-Oz Z, et al. Sole pathogen in acute bronchiolitis: is there a role for other organisms apart from respiratory syncytial virus? Pediatr Infect Dis J 2010;29(1):e7–10.
75. Song JR, Jin Y, Xie ZP, et al. Novel human bocavirus in children with acute respiratory tract infection. Emerg Infect Dis 2010;16(2):324–7.
76. Lu X, Gooding LR, Erdman DD. Human bocavirus in tonsillar lymphocytes. Emerg Infect Dis 2008;14(8):1332–4.
77. Schenk T, Strahm B, Kontny U, et al. Disseminated bocavirus infection after stem cell transplant. Emerg Infect Dis 2007;13(9):1425–7.
78. Dijkman R, Koekkoek SM, Molenkamp R, et al. Human bocavirus can be cultured in differentiated human airway epithelial cells. J Virol 2009;83(15):7739–48.
79. Brieu N, Gay B, Segondy M, et al. Electron microscopy observation of human bocavirus (HBoV) in nasopharyngeal samples from HBoV-infected children. J Clin Microbiol 2007;45(10):3419–20.
80. Arthur JL, Higgins GD, Davidson GP, et al. A novel bocavirus associated with acute gastroenteritis in Australian children. PLoS Pathog 2009;5(4):e1000391.
81. Kapoor A, Slikas E, Simmonds P, et al. A newly identified bocavirus species in human stool. J Infect Dis 2009;199(2):196–200.
82. Calvo C, Pozo F, Garcia-Garcia M, et al. Detection of new respiratory viruses in hospitalized infants with bronchiolitis: a three-year prospective study. Acta Paediatr 2010;99:883–7.
83. Vallet C, Pons-Catalano C, Mandelcwajg A, et al. Human bocavirus: a cause of severe asthma exacerbation in children. J Pediatr 2009;155(2):286–8.
84. Nadji SA, Poos-Ashkan L, Khalilzadeh S, et al. Phylogenetic analysis of human bocavirus isolated from children with acute respiratory illnesses and gastroenteritis in Iran. Scand J Infect Dis 2010;42:598–603.

85. Midulla F, Scagnolari C, Bonci E, et al. Respiratory syncytial virus, human bocavirus and rhinovirus bronchiolitis in infants. Arch Dis Child 2010;95(1):35–41.
86. Allander T, Andreasson K, Gupta S, et al. Identification of a third human polyomavirus. J Virol 2007;81(8):4130–6.
87. Gaynor AM, Nissen MD, Whiley DM, et al. Identification of a novel polyomavirus from patients with acute respiratory tract infections. PLoS Pathog 2007;3(5):e64.
88. Hormozdi DJ, Arens MQ, Le B-M, et al. KI polyomavirus detected in respiratory tract specimens from patients in St. Louis, Missouri. Pediatr Infect Dis J 2010; 29(4):329–33.
89. Mueller A, Simon A, Gillen J, et al. Polyomaviruses KI and WU in children with respiratory tract infection. Arch Virol 2009;154(10):1605–8.
90. Bialasiewicz S, Whiley DM, Lambert SB, et al. Presence of the newly discovered human polyomaviruses KI and WU in Australian patients with acute respiratory tract infection. J Clin Virol 2008;41(2):63–8.
91. Babakir-Mina M, Ciccozzi M, Bonifacio D, et al. Identification of the novel KI and WU polyomaviruses in human tonsils. J Clin Virol 2009;46(1):75–9.
92. Norja P, Ubillos I, Templeton K, et al. No evidence for an association between infections with WU and KI polyomaviruses and respiratory disease. J Clin Virol 2007;40(4):307–11.
93. Imperiale MJ, Major EO. Polyomaviruses. In: Knipe DM, Howley PM, editors. Fields virology, vol. 1. Philadelphia: Lippincott-Raven; 2005. p. 2263–98.
94. Zhao L, Qian Y, Zhu R, et al. Identification of WU polyomavirus from pediatric patients with acute respiratory infections in Beijing, China. Arch Virol 2010; 155(2):181–6.
95. Le B-M, Demertzis LM, Wu G, et al. Clinical and epidemiologic characterization of WU polyomavirus infection, St. Louis, Missouri. Emerg Infect Dis 2007;13(12): 1936–8.
96. Payungporn S, Chieochansin T, Thongmee C, et al. Prevalence and molecular characterization of WU/KI polyomaviruses isolated from pediatric patients with respiratory disease in Thailand. Virus Res 2008;135(2):230–6.
97. Jiang M, Abend JR, Johnson SF, et al. The role of polyomaviruses in human disease. Virology 2009;384(2):266–73.
98. Sharp CP, Norja P, Anthony I, et al. Reactivation and mutation of newly discovered WU, KI, and Merkel cell carcinoma polyomaviruses in immunosuppressed individuals. J Infect Dis 2009;199(3):398–404.
99. Nguyen NL, Le B-M, Wang D. Serologic evidence of frequent human infection with WU and KI polyomaviruses. Emerg Infect Dis 2009;15(8):1199–205.

Animal Models of Virus-induced Chronic Airway Disease

Louis A. Rosenthal, PhD

KEYWORDS

- Viral respiratory tract infections • Asthma • Animal models
- Respiratory tract viruses • Airway dysfunction • Asthma onset

Physicians recognized a link between the common cold and asthma long before the discovery of the viral causation of colds. The great physician-philosopher Moses Maimonides wrote in the twelfth century that with regard to asthma, "I conclude that this disorder starts with a common cold, especially in the rainy season, and the patient is forced to gasp for breath day and night, depending on the duration of the onset, until the phlegm is expelled, the flow completed and the lung well cleared."[1] In 1698, the pioneering English physician and clinical investigator Sir John Floyer, who himself had asthma, stated in his classic work, *A Treatise of the Asthma*, "I cannot remember the first occasion of my asthma; but have been told that it was a cold when I first went to school."[2] Although physicians observed associations between colds and asthma, it is only recently that improved methods of respiratory tract virus detection have permitted intensive investigation of these links and the potential role of early-life viral respiratory tract infections in the inception of asthma.

Despite the growing evidence that experiencing viral wheezing illnesses early in life is an important risk factor for the development of asthma,[3–6] a detailed understanding of the role of these infections in the onset of asthma remains to be elucidated.[7] It seems likely that a complex interplay of viral, host, environmental, and developmental factors influences the processes by which viral respiratory tract infections contribute to asthma inception. A central issue in asthma research is the role that acute insults to the airways, such as viral infections, play in the eventual development of chronic airway abnormalities. Animal models of virus-induced chronic airway dysfunction

This work was supported by grant nos. AI070503 and HL097134 from the National Institutes of Health.

Division of Allergy, Pulmonary and Critical Care Medicine, Department of Medicine, University of Wisconsin School of Medicine and Public Health, 600 Highland Avenue, K4-948 CSC-9988, Madison, WI 53792, USA

E-mail address: lar@medicine.wisc.edu

can serve as important investigative tools to address this issue because they permit control and manipulation of host genetic factors through the use of defined inbred, transgenic, and knockout animal strains and developmental factors through the capacity to perform viral inoculations and evaluate the outcomes of viral respiratory tract infections at specific stages of development. Furthermore, the nature of the airway insult (ie, an infection with a respiratory tract virus) is known, and the animals can be inoculated with respiratory tract viruses in a specific and controlled manner. In this article, the potential advantages and disadvantages of using animal models for investigating the mechanisms by which early-life viral respiratory tract infections could initiate a process leading to chronic airway dysfunction and the asthmatic phenotype are discussed. A variety of useful animal models have been developed to study various aspects of viral respiratory tract infections of relevance to asthma. These models have used a variety of animal species, including mice,[8–15] rats,[16–24] guinea pigs,[25] cotton rats,[26] sheep[27], cattle,[28] and nonhuman primates.[29] This review discusses the potential advantages and disadvantages of models in mice and rats because most work has been performed in these species.

There is increasing evidence that viral wheezing illnesses in early life, especially those caused by infections with human rhinovirus (HRV), are associated with an increased risk of developing asthma in childhood.[3–6] Viral respiratory tract infections also are the main cause of asthma exacerbations in children and adults.[30] In addition, repeated viral respiratory tract infections during childhood might be a factor in the generation of the persistent airway changes associated with asthma.[31] There is also evidence of interaction between early-life viral respiratory tract infections, atopy (the genetic predisposition to produce high levels of IgE in response to allergen exposure), and allergic sensitization (a manifestation of atopy) in relation to the risk for developing asthma. Children who experience viral respiratory tract infections with wheezing in early life and develop allergic sensitization are at substantially greater risk for developing persistent wheezing and childhood asthma than are children who experience one or the other or neither.[3,5] Therefore, there is a strong need for the development of animal models that can mimic these early-life viral respiratory tract infections; in particular, those early-life viral infections that seem to have long-lasting consequences for respiratory health. Consequently, it is important to develop rodent models of asthma that include this feature (ie, an early-life respiratory infection that results in persistent airway sequelae). It would be especially useful if these models also had the capacity to incorporate components of allergic sensitization and allergic airway inflammation, which seem to be important factors in the development of childhood asthma. Because the inception of childhood asthma might depend on interactions between the immune and pulmonary systems in early life, it would be important for the models to have the capacity to examine both the immunologic and physiologic consequences of relevant viral respiratory tract infections. Many of the viral respiratory tract infection models in rodents, although highly useful, have focused on the acute effects of the viral infection and the acute interactions with allergic sensitization and acute allergic airway inflammation. A more limited number of models have also addressed chronic, long-term effects of viral respiratory tract infections in the context of attempting to better understand the origins of asthma.[8–10,16–23]

WHAT MIGHT AN IDEAL RODENT MODEL LOOK LIKE?

To consider the potential advantages and disadvantages of using rodent models to study virus-induced chronic airway dysfunction, it would be useful to consider what features might be incorporated in an ideal model. Recent evidence indicates that viral wheezing illnesses and atopy, as shown by allergic sensitization, may have additive or perhaps even synergistic effects with regard to the associated risk for the development of persistent wheezing and asthma in childhood.[3–6] Therefore, an ideal rodent model would allow investigators to examine important aspects of these interactions from multiple perspectives. The ability to study relevant host genetic factors would be important. For example, it would be of great value to be able to study genetic aspects of atopy and susceptibility to allergic sensitization, as well as genetic factors regulating the susceptibility to viral respiratory tract infections and postviral airway sequelae. The capacity to manipulate environmental factors, such as exposures to respiratory tract viruses and allergens, would be necessary. The ability to investigate developmental factors, such as the effects of the maturational states of the immune and pulmonary systems on the responses to respiratory tract virus and/or allergen exposure and the subsequent development of chronic airway sequelae, would be of great importance as well. Overall, an ideal model of asthma inception would allow for the investigation of mechanisms that could potentially tie together the host immunologic responses to environmental insults to the airways (in this case respiratory tract virus infections), atopy and allergic sensitization, and the subsequent development of persistent structural and functional changes to the airways that might lead to development of the asthmatic phenotype. To further this discussion of the potential advantages and disadvantages of rodent models of virus-induced chronic airway dysfunction, the capacity of these models to investigate relevant viral, host, environmental, and developmental factors is considered.

Viral Factors

Despite the increasing evidence that early-life viral wheezing illnesses are strongly associated with increased risk for the development of persistent wheezing and asthma in childhood, the mechanisms by which viral wheezing illnesses could mediate these affects are poorly understood. In addition, a causal role for these viral wheezing illnesses in the onset of asthma has yet to be established. Viral wheezing illnesses might trigger long-term airway sequelae in susceptible infants and children, leading to the development of asthma. However, it is also possible that infants and children who subsequently go on to develop asthma because of abnormalities in their lungs or immune systems are particularly susceptible to wheezing brought on by viral respiratory tract infections. That is, are viral wheezing illnesses a contributing factor to the development of asthma or are they a marker for individuals who develop asthma for other reasons? Or can both of these scenarios occur in different individuals? Rodent models of virus-induced chronic airway dysfunction could be useful in addressing the relative importance of viral factors as mechanisms by which viral respiratory tract infections could cause chronic structure-function changes in the airways that could lead to long-lasting physiologic abnormalities. These mechanisms could then be tested under the more limited conditions of what can be studied directly in children. That is, rodent studies can yield testable hypotheses that could be investigated in new prospective asthma cohort studies or through the use of banked clinical specimens from previous and ongoing asthma cohort studies. **Box 1** summarizes potential advantages and disadvantages of using rodent models to investigate mechanisms of virus-induced chronic airway dysfunction.

Important unresolved questions include whether specific respiratory tract viruses might be asthmagenic and if so, whether different respiratory tract viruses vary in their asthmagenic potential. That is, are certain viruses more or less likely to cause respiratory tract infections that can trigger the chronic alterations in airway function observed in asthma? Rodent models can provide a useful way to investigate mechanisms by

---

Box 1
Use of rodent models for investigating the role of viral factors in virus-induced chronic airway dysfunction

Potential Advantages

1. The timing of viral inoculations is at the investigator's convenience, permitting reproducible observation of the entire natural history of the respiratory tract virus infection

2. Respiratory tract viruses can be genetically modified before inoculation to identify and characterize viral virulence factors

3. Mechanisms by which viral virulence factors subvert host defenses can be investigated by inoculating rodents with genetic deficiencies in antiviral response pathways

4. A variety of viruses can be directly compared in experimental inoculation studies

5. Useful models can be established by infecting rodents with rodent respiratory tract viruses, which replicate efficiently in rodent airway cells and require lower viral doses to achieve airway infection and inflammation in rodents than do human respiratory tract viruses

6. Models can be useful for preclinical studies of therapeutic interventions and antiviral medications

7. Rodents can be inoculated with emerging respiratory tract viruses, which would be unsafe to do in humans

8. Cells, tissues, and organs are available for analysis of viral titers, viral gene, and protein expression, and expression of viral virulence factors at any time after viral inoculation

Potential Disadvantages

1. Human respiratory tract viruses, when inoculated into rodents, often replicate inefficiently in rodent airway cells and require high viral doses to achieve airway infection and inflammation

2. Rodents might not express a receptor for the human respiratory tract virus

3. Viral virulence factors might operate differently in rodents than in humans because of host-related differences in antiviral responses

---

which respiratory tract viruses vary in their asthmagenic potential. For example, investigators have shown that different strains of respiratory syncytial virus (RSV) can differ in their pathogenicity and ability to induce mucus production in a well-defined mouse model.[32] These investigators have been able to define genetic differences among these RSV strains that account for this diversity in mucogenicity and pathogenicity.

An important issue with regard to rodent models of viral respiratory tract infections is the permissiveness of the host for the virus of interest. Some of the advantages and disadvantages of these rodent models can be a consequence of which respiratory tract virus is used in the model. For example, an advantage of the recent establishment of mouse models of HRV infection is that these models use one of the viruses that cause HRV infections and illnesses in humans.[33,34] The disadvantage is that HRV does not replicate as efficiently in mice as it does in the human host. Consequently, high doses of HRV must be used to establish transient infections in the mice.[33,34] Even although the replication of HRV in mice is limited, these models continue to be useful for studying the mechanisms of HRV-induced inflammation.[33,34] A mouse-adapted strain of HRV has been generated in vitro,[35] and it would be interesting to see if this virus replicates more efficiently in mice than nonadapted HRV strains. Because there are no known rodent rhinoviruses, we have used a related rodent picornavirus (HRV is a member of the picornavirus family), mengovirus, to establish respiratory infection models in rats[36] and mice (LA Rosenthal, unpublished data, 2010), which has the advantage of using a natural rodent virus in a natural host. Therefore, the required viral dose is smaller and viral shedding occurs for a longer time than in the HRV infection model in mice.[36] Rodent models using rodent parainfluenza 1 (Sendai) virus, which like RSV is also a paramyxovirus, have been particularly useful because this virus replicates well in the rodent host and more closely resembles a natural virus exposure.[8–10,16–23] A potential disadvantage to consider when using rodent respiratory tract viruses is that they might exhibit differences with regard to viral virulence mechanisms compared with the corresponding human respiratory tract viruses.

Another important consideration with regard to viral factors is the so-called hit-and-run hypothesis.[37] That is, it is hypothesized that a viral respiratory tract infection occurs early in life and even after the virus has been cleared by the host, an array of processes have been set in motion that lead to long-term airway sequelae that are dependent on the initiating viral infection. It is likely that the viral respiratory tract infection must be moderate to severe and involve the lower airways for it to have significant enough effects to set such a process in motion (ie, the virus would have induced a spectrum of disorders ranging from wheezing illnesses to bronchiolitis). How a single respiratory tract virus infection could have such long-lasting consequences remains to be elucidated, but rodent models of virus-induced chronic airway dysfunction are providing an important path for investigating this possibility and the mechanisms that could contribute to this process.[8–10,16–23] The results from these rodent models can inform the design of studies in humans, allowing the hypotheses generated from the animal model data to be tested in human clinical studies. The hit-and-run hypothesis remains a viable one, and an ideal rodent model of virus-induced chronic airway dysfunction would almost certainly have characteristics that would enable the investigation of this hypothesis. Two rodent models studying the postviral airway sequelae following Sendai virus bronchiolitis have been useful for looking at these questions[8–10,16–23] and have directly led to new hypotheses and to studies in humans to test them.[10,38]

The binding specificity of human respiratory tract viruses for their cellular receptors is also an important consideration and a potential disadvantage when designing rodent models of viral respiratory tract infection. Differences in receptor-binding capacity to rodent cells can limit the ability of human respiratory tract viruses to be studied in rodent models (ie, the human virus is unable to bind to and enter rodent host cells). A notable example is the inability of major group HRV to infect rodent cells because of the requirement for binding to intercellular adhesion molecule 1 (ICAM-1).[35] HRV cannot use murine ICAM 1 for entry into cells. This difficulty has been overcome in one model by using transgenic mice that constitutively express human ICAM-1 as the host for inoculation with a major group HRV.[33] Thus, one advantage of using rodent respiratory tract viruses in the design of rodent models of virus-induced chronic airway dysfunction is that the virus and its receptor are compatible.

Another distinct advantage of rodent models is that the entire progression of the viral infection can be observed because the initiation of the viral infection is controlled by the investigator. Thus, in rodent models all stages of the viral respiratory tract infection as well as any sequelae identified during the chronic phase after the clearance of the virus can be studied. In addition, cells, tissues, and organs from the immune and pulmonary systems of rodents are readily available for analysis of viral titers, viral gene and protein expression, and the expression of viral virulence factors at any time after inoculation with the respiratory tract virus.

In studies involving humans, the only instance when this is true is in experimental inoculation studies, which are of great value but are technically challenging, and few research centers have the capacity to perform them. Otherwise, most human studies involve individuals who present with viral respiratory tract infections. Even in large cohort studies where individuals are monitored prospectively, infections become apparent only when presented to the investigators by the individuals or their parents/caregivers in the case of infants and children. A potential disadvantage in rodent models is that the course of infection in rodents is unlikely to be identical to that in humans (eg, the kinetics are likely to be somewhat different). Also, most inoculations of rodents deposit the virus both in the nasopharynx and the lungs, whereas the initiation of viral respiratory tract infections with typical cold viruses in humans is more likely to occur with deposition of virus in the nose and/or eyes, which then infects the lower airways.

In rodent models, it is possible to administer respiratory tract viruses that have been genetically modified to investigate viral virulence factors. In experimental inoculations of humans this procedure would not usually be possible, with the exception of inoculation with experimental or approved vaccine strains of reduced virulence. Inoculation of humans with respiratory tract viruses that have been genetically modified to increase virulence is not ethically acceptable. However, this procedure would be possible in rodent models if appropriate precautions were taken and appropriate containment procedures were used.

When new respiratory tract viruses of potential relevance to asthma are discovered, it is possible to attempt experimental inoculations of rodents immediately if stocks can be prepared; a notable example is the rapid development of mouse models of metapneumovirus-induced respiratory infection.[39,40] In contrast, experimental inoculations of humans would involve a long safety testing and regulatory process, including an investigational new drug application to the US Food and Drug Administration, and may not be ethically possible depending on the virulence of the virus in humans. In addition, clinical respiratory tract virus challenges in humans require a large infrastructure of investigators, research coordinators, and laboratory personnel and few research centers have the capacity to do this.

An instructive example of the ability of rodent models to be useful for the investigation of viral factors involves the recent advance in understanding the important association between HRV-induced wheezing illnesses and the development of childhood asthma. HRV had been implicated as the most common viral infection associated with asthma exacerbations in children and adults.[30] However, recent birth cohort studies in the United States and Australia have also shown that HRV infections are a significant cause of wheezing illnesses in infants and children and that these HRV wheezing illnesses are associated with an increased risk for the development of asthma in childhood, especially if the children are sensitized to allergen.[3–6] Because viral challenge studies, even with safety-tested strains of HRV, are not feasible in children, rodent models provide an avenue for investigating the effects of HRV in younger animals to model what may be happening in infants and children.

The available animal models include those using minor group HRV, which binds to the low-density lipoprotein receptor on both human and rodent cells,[33,34] those using major group HRV, which binds to ICAM-1,[33] requiring the use of mice transgenic for human ICAM-1 because HRV does not bind to mouse ICAM-1, and our use of a related murine picornavirus, mengovirus, to model HRV infections.[36] All of the published studies have used young adult rodents for the development of these models. Inoculation experiments on young adult animals provide data that are relevant to colds and cold virus-induced asthma exacerbations. However, it is likely that investigators could take advantage of these novel models to examine effects on younger rodents.

Rodent models also can be advantageous for preclinical testing of novel antiviral therapeutic strategies and for investigating the mechanisms of action of these therapies.[41] However, a caveat is that the viral virulence factors targeted by these therapeutics might differ in rodents compared with those in humans.

Host Factors

Host factors are a crucial consideration in understanding the potential basis for the development of chronic airway dysfunction as a consequence of early-life viral respiratory tract infections. The use of rodent models provides a variety of potential advantages and disadvantages in this regard (**Box 2**). One distinct advantage is that the genetics of the rodent models can be controlled and manipulated to facilitate mechanistic studies. The use of inbred rodent strains dramatically reduces the genetic variability of the experimental subjects. Sophisticated breeding strategies are available that could be used for mapping and characterizing genetic loci associated with host responses to viral respiratory infections.[42] The availability of knockout mouse strains, and the recent but more limited availability of knockout rat strains, enables studies of subjects with specific genetic deficiencies, permitting examination of the effects of specific genes on these processes. In addition, the use of transgenic tools has permitted the development of rodents constitutively expressing or overexpressing genes of potential interest. Of even greater potential value is the development of mouse models in which genes of interest are either conditionally knocked out or expressed, which markedly increases the ability of researchers to control the experimental conditions.[43] A further refinement of these methods has permitted investigators to conditionally knock out or express genes in a cell- or tissue-specific manner through use of cell- and tissue-specific promoters in the constructs that are introduced into the mouse lines. Thus, investigators are able to derive mice that at a time of their choosing can be triggered to knock out, downregulate, or turn on the expression of specific genes of interest, and are able to control the cell specificity,

---

Box 2
Use of rodent models for investigating the role of host factors in virus-induced chronic airway dysfunction

Potential Advantages

1. Use of inbred rodents for viral inoculation studies reduces host genetic variability

2. Use of knockout and transgenic rodent strains for viral inoculation studies facilitates the investigation of the roles of specific host genes in responses to viral respiratory infections

3. Specialized breeding strategies can be used to map and characterize genetic loci associated with host responses to viral respiratory infections

4. The role of atopy in host responses to viral respiratory infections can be investigated by performing viral inoculations in inbred rodent strains that differ in this regard or in knockout or transgenic strains with genetic modifications that influence atopy

5. Cells, tissues, and organs are available for analysis at any time after viral inoculation

Potential Disadvantages

1. There are differences in airway structure/function and physiology between rodents and humans

2. The antiviral responses of rodents and humans are similar but not identical

3. The immune systems of rodents and humans have significant differences

tissue specificity, and the temporal specificity of this modulation of gene expression. That is, investigators are increasingly capable of controlling the levels, location, and timing of gene expression in these models. Transgenic technology also allows investigators to label and track specific cell types and cell subtypes in vivo by expressing fluorescent marker proteins via appropriate promoters with appropriate cell or tissue specificities,[44] which enables cell-tracking experiments that attempt to define the mechanisms regulating the host responses to viral respiratory tract infections.

Another important aspect of host factors that can be studied advantageously in rodent models is the role of gender. Studies can be readily performed in males and females and the results compared and contrasted. This capacity is of importance because of the evidence of gender-related differences in wheezing and asthma in childhood.[45] Rodent models can investigate these issues in a mechanistic way and generate hypotheses to be tested in human studies. In addition, rodent studies can be designed to investigate the mechanisms of gender-related differences observed in human clinical studies.

Another important area of investigation that is becoming amenable to study in rodent models is epigenetic effects, which include heritable changes in gene expression without changes to the underlying genomic sequence.[46,47] The use of rodent models to study the role of epigenetic effects in regulating gene expression during host responses to viral respiratory tract infections would be advantageous because it is possible to modulate epigenetic-relevant DNA modifications through pharmacologic methods. It would also be of interest to investigate whether long-term changes in airways after early-life viral respiratory tract infections could be due in part to epigenetic modifications induced during the host response to the viral infection. The well-established rat and mouse models of Sendai virus-induced chronic airway dysfunction would be attractive candidates for this type of investigation because airway dysfunction in these models continues to persist for the entire period of observation, up to 1 year after viral clearance.[8–10,16–23] Therefore, it likely that the persistent airway inflammation and dysfunction are caused by host factors that were initiated by the viral infection and then persisted even after viral clearance (ie, the hit-and-run hypothesis). If epigenetic effects could be defined in these rodent models, focused hypotheses could be generated for testing in human studies using the more limited array of biologic samples that can be obtained from infants and children enrolled in prospective cohort studies.

Rodent models also can play an important role in addressing the mechanistic role of atopy, the genetic predisposition to produce high levels of IgE in response to allergen exposure, in the development of virus-induced chronic airway dysfunction. Rodent strains differ with regard to their capacity to generate IgE and Th2-type immune responses, which is useful for investigating the interaction of viral respiratory tract infections and subsequent antiviral host responses with the atopic status of the host. This characteristic has been an important aspect of the Brown Norway rat (BN) model of virus-induced chronic airway dysfunction, in which only rats of the atopic BN strain are susceptible to the development of a postbronchiolitis, asthmalike phenotype after experiencing parainfluenza 1 (Sendai) virus-induced bronchiolitis as weanlings. F344 rats, after undergoing the same viral inoculation under the same conditions, experience a resolution of the viral bronchiolitis and have normal airways after several weeks.[16–23,48] One significant difference between these strains is their atopic status. The BN rat has Th2-biased immune responses, whereas the F344 rat mounts Th1-biased immune responses. BN rats can make substantial amounts of IgE after allergen sensitization, whereas it is difficult to generate IgE responses in F344 rats. Although these global differences in the ability to mount the Th2-type responses that promote allergic inflammation are useful, transgenic and knockout rodents permit even finer distinctions with regard to atopy to be investigated: the effects of individual genes can be investigated with regard to their effects on suscep- tibility to allergic sensitization and the subsequent development of allergic inflamma- tion. Information derived from these studies can then inform studies in humans in which genes identified in rodent models can be investigated (eg, by examining asso- ciations between genetic polymorphisms in these genes of interest and the develop- ment of allergic sensitization and asthma, as well as how they influence susceptibility to the early-life viral respiratory tract infections that might contribute to the develop- ment of chronic airway dysfunction).

Another issue to consider is that there are notable differences in pulmonary physi- ology between rodents and humans.[49] For example, the airway caliber in rodents, especially in mice, is larger relative to their body size compared with humans. This is one reason why it can be difficult to detect airway obstruction in mice with viral respiratory tract infections in the absence of a challenge with a cholinergic agent, such as methacholine. These rodent models are still useful, but it is important to keep these differences in mind when interpreting physiology data from rodent models of human airway disease.

Environmental Factors

Rodent models present both potential advantages and disadvantages with regard to the investigation of the influences of environmental factors on host responses to viral respiratory tract infections and the development of chronic airway dysfunction (**Box 3**). One advantage is that it is possible to design controlled exposures to defined environ- mental factors, such as microorganisms, microbial products (eg, endotoxin, microbial DNA, glucans), dusts, allergens, diesel exhaust, ozone, and tobacco smoke and then assess how these exposures affect the responses of the rodents to a challenge with

---

Box 3
Use of rodent models for investigating the role of environmental factors in virus-induced chronic airway dysfunction

Potential Advantages

1. Timing, dose, and frequency of environmental exposures that are being tested for their ability to modulate host responses to viral respiratory tract infections can be controlled

2. Gene-by-environment interactions that might influence host responses to viral respiratory tract infections can be studied under conditions in which both the environmental and host genetic factors are controlled

3. Prenatal and postnatal environmental exposures can be performed in a controlled manner

4. Cells, tissues, and organs are available for analysis at any time during and after environmental exposures and viral inoculations

Potential Disadvantages

1. In rodent models, it can be difficult to replicate the complexity of the environmental factors encountered by humans

2. The time frame of rodent studies often dictates that the timing of environmental exposures is accelerated and that higher doses of environmental agents are required to generate biologic effects

3. Rodents and humans might respond differently to environmental exposures

a respiratory tract virus. That is, do these environmental exposures act as comorbid factors to increase the likelihood of developing or the severity of virus-induced chronic airway dysfunction? Alternatively, do these environmental exposures boost the capacity of the host to resolve the viral challenge in a way that prevents the development of chronic airway dysfunction? It is also advantageous that exposures can be made during specific developmental windows encompassing different maturational stages of the immune system and lungs. Defined prenatal and/or postnatal exposures can be performed as well to study in utero effects. Foster nursing approaches can be used to investigate effects of breast milk consumption.

The dose, frequency, and duration of the exposures can be controlled and quantified. This strategy has been shown to be important, for example, with regard to the effects of environmental exposures to microbial products, such as endotoxin. Studies in rodent models and epidemiologic studies in humans have shown substantial dosage effects in which lower levels of exposure may increase the risk of allergen sensitization, whereas higher levels of exposure may have protective effects in this regard.[50,51] This situation is further complicated by interactions with host factors, especially the genetics of the host, whereby gene-by-environment interactions can modulate the effect of exposures to microbial products (eg, endotoxin).[51] The use of rodent models can permit detailed mechanistic studies of these types of gene-by-environment interactions through the use of knockout mice or transgenic mice overexpressing the genes of interest and by the ability to perform prospective dose-response experiments. A disadvantage of rodent models is that the environmental exposures are not so complex as those in the human environment; therefore, important interactive effects among different types of environmental exposures might not be appreciated. To address this issue there has been interest among some investigators in taking a less reductionist approach and exposing the rodent to more complex mixtures, such as house dust extracts.[52] It seems likely that both approaches, exposure to one or 2 specific environmental agents versus exposure to more complex mixtures of environmental agents, yield complementary findings that inform each other.

Another issue to consider is the differences in dosages and timing of environmental exposures between rodent models and the experiences of humans. One of the major values of using rodents as research models is that their short life span permits contraction of the time that would be required to perform similar studies in humans. However, this strategy often results in the need for a more compressed schedule of exposures with larger amounts of material to achieve effects that can be studied in these shorter time frames. Thus, it is important for the research community to periodically assess the relevance of rodent models by comparing data from rodents and humans and to use data from clinical research to design novel mechanistic studies in rodent models and vice versa to use mechanistic studies in rodents to suggest hypotheses to be tested in clinically oriented studies.

The difficulty of exposing rodents to the complexity of environmental factors encountered by humans is being alleviated by the development of new technologies that permit the characterization of this complexity. This strategy allows investigators to replicate aspects of these complex environmental exposures to study potential interactive effects within their rodent models of virus-induced airway dysfunction. For example, multiplex technologies have been developed that can assay for multiple allergens within environmental samples.[53] The development of microarray technologies to detect practically all known bacterial species allows the careful delineation of bacterial species within different environments,[54] such as farming environments, that could have an effect on the outcome of early-life viral respiratory tract infections.

This process allows investigators to better define how these complex mixtures can affect the development of host antiviral responses, the characteristics of which may have profound effects on the likelihood that chronic airway sequelae develop after a viral respiratory tract infection in early life.

Developmental Factors

Rodent models of virus-induced airway dysfunction also exhibit advantages and disadvantages with regard to studying developmental factors (**Box 4**). A major advantage is the shorter life span of the rodent, which enables longitudinal studies encompassing all ages to be performed within a convenient period. These types of longitudinal studies are also performed in humans but require large teams of investigators working for many years. Although these pediatric cohort studies are invaluable, the rodent models permit similar questions to be addressed in a mechanistic manner in a condensed time frame. The data derived from these rodent studies can then be used to generate focused hypotheses to be addressed in clinical studies. A disadvantage of rodent models is that harmonizing human and rodent maturational stages with regard to the immune system and pulmonary system can present some challenges. For example, in rodents alveolarization occurs postnatally; rodent pups are born with saccules. Therefore, respiratory viral challenges must take this into account. For example, Sendai virus infection of neonatal rats yielded an interesting model,[55] but it was unsatisfactory for the kinds of changes associated with the development of asthma because it induced alveolar dysplasia (ie, the viral infection interfered with the normal course of postnatal alveolar development, which in humans would have occurred prenatally). Thus, the BN rat model of the postbronchiolitis, asthmalike phenotype was developed by infecting weanling (3- to 4-week-old) BN rats with Sendai virus, which induced bronchiolitis without alveolar dysplasia, because alveolarization had already occurred in these weanling animals.[16–23]

Box 4
Use of rodent models for investigating the role of developmental factors in virus-induced chronic airway dysfunction

Potential Advantages

1. Shorter lifespan of rodents allows study of chronic postviral airway sequelae within a convenient period

2. The developmental window in which viral inoculations are performed can be chosen

3. Cells, tissues, and organs are available for analysis at any age

4. Knockout and transgenic rodent strains can receive viral inoculations at any age to define the effect of specific genes on developmental factors regulating host responses to viral respiratory tract infections

Potential Disadvantages

1. Prenatal and postnatal developmental progress is scaled differently in rodents compared with humans

2. There are differences in prenatal and postnatal lung maturation between rodents and humans

3. There are differences in the prenatal and postnatal maturation of the immune system between rodents and humans

An important aspect of rodent models is the ability to perform manipulations prenatally as well as postnatally under defined conditions. For example, this procedure can help to distinguish in utero influences from other effects. With the growing interest in regulatory mechanisms such as epigenetics, investigation of in utero effects is likely to become an important area of research.

The availability of knockout and transgenic rodent strains allows investigators to look at the effects of specific genes during development on the response to viral respiratory tract infections. Although these studies do not replace pediatric clinical studies, they permit a mechanistic focus and are complementary to studies involving humans.

Another advantage of developmental studies in rodents is the capability to sample cells and tissues. Many cell and tissue samples are difficult to obtain from children because of ethical, safety, and logistical reasons. For example, the ability to obtain approvals for experimental bronchoscopy of children is markedly different in the different regions of the world and even at different institutions within the same country. The ability to perform these types of procedures ranges from almost never to sometimes with sufficient justification. The tissue availability from the rodent models does provide the capacity to perform certain types of mechanistic studies that cannot be performed in children. These mechanistic studies can then serve as a basis for designing focused studies in pediatric subjects when access to biologic samples can be limited and the amount of material in the samples can also be limiting.

REFERENCES

1. Maimonides M. Treatise on asthma. In: Muntner S, editor. Medical writings of Moses Maimonides. Philadelphia: Lippincott; 1963. p. 2.
2. Floyer J. A treatise of the asthma. London: Richard Wilkin; 1698.
3. Kusel MM, de Klerk NH, Kebadze T, et al. Early-life respiratory viral infections, atopic sensitization, and risk of subsequent development of persistent asthma. J Allergy Clin Immunol 2007;119(5):1105–10.
4. Lemanske RF Jr, Jackson DJ, Gangnon RE, et al. Rhinovirus illnesses during infancy predict subsequent childhood wheezing. J Allergy Clin Immunol 2005; 116(3):571–7.
5. Jackson DJ, Gangnon RE, Evans MD, et al. Wheezing rhinovirus illnesses in early life predict asthma development in high-risk children. Am J Respir Crit Care Med 2008;178(7):667–72.
6. Sly PD, Kusel M, Holt PG. Do early-life viral infections cause asthma? J Allergy Clin Immunol 2010;125(6):1202–5.
7. Rosenthal LA, Avila PC, Heymann PW, et al. Viral respiratory tract infections and asthma: the course ahead. J Allergy Clin Immunol 2010;125(6):1212–7.
8. Walter MJ, Morton JD, Kajiwara N, et al. Viral induction of a chronic asthma phenotype and genetic segregation from the acute response. J Clin Invest 2002;110(2):165–75.
9. Grayson MH, Cheung D, Rohlfing MM, et al. Induction of high-affinity IgE receptor on lung dendritic cells during viral infection leads to mucous cell metaplasia. J Exp Med 2007;204(11):2759–69.
10. Kim EY, Battaile JT, Patel AC, et al. Persistent activation of an innate immune response translates respiratory viral infection into chronic lung disease. Nat Med 2008;14(6):633–40.
11. Matsuse H, Behera AK, Kumar M, et al. Recurrent respiratory syncytial virus infections in allergen-sensitized mice lead to persistent airway inflammation and hyperresponsiveness. J Immunol 2000;164(12):6583–92.

12. Hashimoto K, Graham BS, Ho SB, et al. Respiratory syncytial virus in allergic lung inflammation increases muc5ac and gob-5. Am J Respir Crit Care Med 2004; 170(3):306–12.
13. Hashimoto K, Durbin JE, Zhou W, et al. Respiratory syncytial virus infection in the absence of STAT1 results in airway dysfunction, airway mucus, and augmented IL-17 levels. J Allergy Clin Immunol 2005;116(3):550–7.
14. Estripeaut D, Torres JP, Somers CS, et al. Respiratory syncytial virus persistence in the lungs correlates with airway hyperreactivity in the mouse model. J Infect Dis 2008;198(10):1435–43.
15. Mejias A, Chavez-Bueno S, Gomez AM, et al. Respiratory syncytial virus persistence: evidence in the mouse model. Pediatr Infect Dis J 2008;27(Suppl 10):S60–2.
16. Rosenthal LA, Sorkness RL, Lemanske RF Jr. Origin of respiratory virus-induced chronic airway dysfunction: exploring genetic, developmental, and environmental factors in a rat model of the asthmatic phenotype. In: Johnston SL, Papadopoulos NG, editors, Respiratory infections in allergy and asthma lung biology in health and disease, vol. 178. New York: Marcel Dekker; 2003. p. 365–88.
17. Uhl EW, Castleman WL, Sorkness RL, et al. Parainfluenza virus-induced persistence of airway inflammation, fibrosis, and dysfunction associated with TGF-β_1 expression in Brown Norway rats. Am J Respir Crit Care Med 1996;154:1834–42.
18. Kumar A, Sorkness R, Kaplan MR, et al. Chronic, episodic, reversible airway obstruction after viral bronchiolitis in rats. Am J Respir Crit Care Med 1997;155: 130–4.
19. Sorkness RL, Castleman WL, Kumar A, et al. Prevention of chronic post-bronchiolitis airway sequelae with interferon-γ treatment in rats. Am J Respir Crit Care Med 1999;160:705–10.
20. Sorkness RL, Gern JE, Grindle KA, et al. Persistence of viral RNA in 2 rat strains differing in susceptibility to postbronchiolitis airway dysfunction. J Allergy Clin Immunol 2002;110(4):607–9.
21. Sorkness RL, Tuffaha A. Contribution of airway closure to chronic postbronchiolitis airway dysfunction in rats. J Appl Physiol 2004;96(3):904–10.
22. Rosenthal LA, Mikus LD, Tuffaha A, et al. Attenuated innate mechanisms of interferon-γ production in rats susceptible to postviral airway dysfunction. Am J Respir Cell Mol Biol 2004;30(5):702–9.
23. Sorkness RL, Herricks KM, Szakaly RJ, et al. Altered allergen-induced eosinophil trafficking and physiological dysfunction in airways with preexisting virus-induced injury. Am J Physiol Lung Cell Mol Physiol 2007;292(1):L85–91.
24. Piedimonte G, Hegele RG, Auais A. Persistent airway inflammation after resolution of respiratory syncytial virus infection in rats. Pediatr Res 2004;55(4):657–65.
25. Adamko DJ, Yost BL, Gleich GJ, et al. Ovalbumin sensitization changes the inflammatory response to subsequent parainfluenza infection. Eosinophils mediate airway hyperresponsiveness, m(2) muscarinic receptor dysfunction, and antiviral effects. J Exp Med 1999;190(10):1465–78.
26. Hassantoufighi A, Oglesbee M, Richter BW, et al. Respiratory syncytial virus replication is prolonged by a concomitant allergic response. Clin Exp Immunol 2007; 148(2):218–29.
27. Olivier A, Gallup J, de Macedo MM, et al. Human respiratory syncytial virus A2 strain replicates and induces innate immune responses by respiratory epithelia of neonatal lambs. Int J Exp Pathol 2009;90(4):431–8.
28. Gershwin LJ, Gunther RA, Hornof WJ, et al. Effect of infection with bovine respiratory syncytial virus on pulmonary clearance of an inhaled antigen in calves. Am J Vet Res 2008;69(3):416–22.

29. Mohapatra SS, Boyapalle S. Epidemiologic, experimental, and clinical links between respiratory syncytial virus infection and asthma. Clin Microbiol Rev 2008;21(3):495–504.

30. Friedlander SL, Busse WW. The role of rhinovirus in asthma exacerbations. J Allergy Clin Immunol 2005;116(2):267–73.

31. Jartti T, Lee WM, Pappas T, et al. Serial viral infections in infants with recurrent respiratory illnesses. Eur Respir J 2008;32(2):314–20.

32. Moore ML, Chi MH, Luongo C, et al. A chimeric A2 strain of respiratory syncytial virus (RSV) with the fusion protein of RSV strain line 19 exhibits enhanced viral load, mucus, and airway dysfunction. J Virol 2009;83(9):4185–94.

33. Bartlett NW, Walton RP, Edwards MR, et al. Mouse models of rhinovirus-induced disease and exacerbation of allergic airway inflammation. Nat Med 2008;14(2): 199–204.

34. Newcomb DC, Sajjan US, Nagarkar DR, et al. Human rhinovirus 1B exposure induces phosphatidylinositol 3-kinase-dependent airway inflammation in mice. Am J Respir Crit Care Med 2008;177(10):1111–21.

35. Harris JR, Racaniello VR. Amino acid changes in proteins 2B and 3A mediate rhinovirus type 39 growth in mouse cells. J Virol 2005;79(9):5363–73.

36. Rosenthal LA, Amineva SP, Szakaly RJ, et al. A rat model of picornavirus-induced airway infection and inflammation. Virol J 2009;6(1):122.

37. Holtzman MJ, Shornick LP, Grayson MH, et al. "Hit-and-run" effects of paramyxoviruses as a basis for chronic respiratory disease. Pediatr Infect Dis J 2004;23(Suppl 11):S235–45.

38. Lemanske RF Jr. The childhood origins of asthma (COAST) study. Pediatr Allergy Immunol 2002;13(Suppl):1538–43.

39. Williams JV, Crowe JE Jr, Enriquez R, et al. Human metapneumovirus infection plays an etiologic role in acute asthma exacerbations requiring hospitalization in adults. J Infect Dis 2005;192(7):1149–53.

40. Guerrero-Plata A, Baron S, Poast JS, et al. Activity and regulation of alpha interferon in respiratory syncytial virus and human metapneumovirus experimental infections. J Virol 2005;79(16):10190–9.

41. Kong X, Zhang W, Lockey RF, et al. Respiratory syncytial virus infection in Fischer 344 rats is attenuated by short interfering RNA against the RSV-NS1 gene. Genet Vaccines Ther 2007;5:4.

42. Flint J, Valdar W, Shifman S, et al. Strategies for mapping and cloning quantitative trait genes in rodents. Nat Rev Genet 2005;6(4):271–86.

43. Hausding M, Sauer K, Maxeiner JH, et al. Transgenic models in allergic responses. Curr Drug Targets 2008;9(6):503–10.

44. Mohrs K, Wakil AE, Killeen N, et al. A two-step process for cytokine production revealed by IL-4 dual-reporter mice. Immunity 2005;23(4):419–29.

45. Lemanske RF Jr, Busse WW. Asthma: clinical expression and molecular mechanisms. J Allergy Clin Immunol 2010;125(2 Suppl 2):S95–102.

46. Holgate ST, Davies DE, Powell RM, et al. Local genetic and environmental factors in asthma disease pathogenesis: chronicity and persistence mechanisms. Eur Respir J 2007;29(4):793–803.

47. Barnes PJ. Targeting the epigenome in the treatment of asthma and chronic obstructive pulmonary disease. Proc Am Thorac Soc 2009;6(8):693–6.

48. Sorkness RL, Castleman WL, Mikus LD, et al. Chronic postbronchiolitis airway instability induced with anti-IFN-gamma antibody in F344 rats. Pediatr Res 2002;52(3):382–6.

49. Bates JH, Rincon M, Irvin CG. Animal models of asthma. Am J Physiol Lung Cell Mol Physiol 2009;297(3):L401–10.

50. Eisenbarth SC, Piggott DA, Huleatt JW, et al. Lipopolysaccharide-enhanced, toll-like receptor 4-dependent T helper cell type 2 responses to inhaled antigen. J Exp Med 2002;196(12):1645–51.

51. Martinez FD. CD14, endotoxin, and asthma risk: actions and interactions. Proc Am Thorac Soc 2007;4(3):221–5.

52. Lam D, Ng N, Lee S, et al. Airway house dust extract exposures modify allergen-induced airway hypersensitivity responses by TLR4-dependent and independent pathways. J Immunol 2008;181(4):2925–32.

53. Earle CD, King EM, Tsay A, et al. High-throughput fluorescent multiplex array for indoor allergen exposure assessment. J Allergy Clin Immunol 2007;119(2): 428–33.

54. DeSantis TZ, Dubosarskiy I, Murray SR, et al. Comprehensive aligned sequence construction for automated design of effective probes (CASCADE-P) using 16S rDNA. Bioinformatics 2003;19(12):1461–8.

55. Castleman WL, Sorkness RL, Lemanske RF Jr, et al. Neonatal viral bronchiolitis and pneumonia induce bronchiolar hypoplasia and alveolar dysplasia in rats. Lab Invest 1988;59:387–96.

The Role of Respiratory Virus Infections in Childhood Asthma Inception

Daniel J. Jackson, MD[a],*, Robert F. Lemanske Jr, MD[a,b]

KEYWORDS

- Human rhinovirus • Respiratory syncytial virus • Wheezing
- Asthma • Children • Interferons

Viral respiratory illnesses associated with wheezing are extremely common during early life and remain a frequent cause of morbidity and hospitalization in young children.[1] Although many children who wheeze with respiratory viruses during infancy outgrow the problem, most children with asthma and reductions in lung function at school age begin wheezing during the first several years of life.[2] Whether symptomatic viral infections of the lower respiratory tract are causal in asthma development or simply identify predisposed children remains a controversial issue. Wheezing illnesses caused by respiratory syncytial virus (RSV), particularly those severe enough to lead to hospitalization, have historically been associated with an increased risk of asthma at school age.[3,4] However, with the development of molecular diagnostics, human rhinovirus (HRV) wheezing illnesses have been recognized more recently as a stronger predictor of school-age asthma than RSV.[5,6] In this article, the authors review the impact of virus infections during early life, focusing primarily on RSV and HRV, and their potential roles in asthma inception.

EPIDEMIOLOGY OF WHEEZING DURING EARLY LIFE

Infections with respiratory viruses are the leading cause of wheezing during early childhood. In fact, with current molecular diagnostics, a viral pathogen can be

Supported by NIH grants 1UL1RR025011, T32 AI007635, P01 HL70831, and by the AAAAI/GSK Allergy Fellow Career Development Award.

[a] Department of Pediatrics, University of Wisconsin School of Medicine and Public Health, 600 Highland Avenue, Madison, WI 53792, USA

[b] Department of Medicine, University of Wisconsin School of Medicine and Public Health, 600 Highland Avenue, Madison, WI 53792, USA

* Corresponding author. Division of Allergy, Immunology, and Rheumatology, University of Wisconsin School of Medicine and Public Health, 600 Highland Avenue CSC H4/468, Madison, WI 53792.

E-mail address: djj@medicine.wisc.edu

identified in at least 90% of wheezing episodes during the first several years of life.[6] All children are infected with respiratory viruses during early life, and up to 50% have a lower respiratory tract illness with wheezing at least once before school age.[2] Several environmental factors have been linked to risk of wheezing illnesses during early life. The Tucson Children's Respiratory Study (TCRS), a prospective unselected birth cohort, identified several risk factors for wheezing during early childhood. Older siblings and daycare, both associated with increased exposure to respiratory viruses, and tobacco smoke exposure were associated with increased risk of early-life wheezing illnesses, whereas breastfeeding was protective.[7]

The most common viruses identified during early-life wheezing illnesses are RSV, HRV, and multiple viruses. Less common causes include parainfluenza, metapneumovirus, coronavirus, influenza, bocavirus, and adenovirus.

RSV is seasonal, with peak infection during winter in the United States. RSV is ubiquitous, with nearly all children infected by 2 years of age.[8] A subset of these children has more severe illnesses, and infection with RSV leading to bronchiolitis and/or pneumonia is a primary cause of hospitalization during the first year of life. Children hospitalized with RSV tend to be younger than children hospitalized for other respiratory viruses. Other risk factors of RSV hospitalization include prematurity, male gender, daycare attendance, and tobacco exposure.[9]

In contrast to RSV, HRV infections occur throughout the year. HRV is the leading cause of bronchiolitis leading to hospitalization in infants outside of the winter bronchiolitis season.[10] Compared with RSV, children hospitalized with HRV tend to be older and are more likely to have wheezed previously.[11] They also often have more atopic risk factors or characteristics, including eczema, allergic sensitization, and parental asthma.

Traditionally, HRVs have been divided into 2 groups (A and B) with about 100 known serotypes. Many HRVs do not grow well in traditional cell culture, and this is particularly true of a novel group of HRVs categorized as Group C HRVs. Molecular diagnostics and characterization of HRVs have demonstrated that the number of HRV species has previously been dramatically underestimated.[12] In fact, numerous recent reports have identified novel Group C HRVs and implicated them in upper and lower respiratory tract illnesses, frequently including illnesses severe enough to lead to hospitalization.[12–16]

VIRUS INFECTION AND SUBSEQUENT ASTHMA DEVELOPMENT
The Role of RSV in Asthma

RSV lower respiratory tract illnesses, particularly those severe enough to lead to hospitalization, are associated with an increased risk of asthma at school age.[3,4] This observation has prompted the idea that RSV lower respiratory tract illness may be causal in asthma development. Sigurs and colleagues[4] used a case-control methodology to examine the risk of asthma and allergy development after RSV bronchiolitis severe enough to lead to hospitalization. They found that severe RSV bronchiolitis was associated with a significantly increased risk of asthma and allergy at 13 years of age, although some have suggested that the rate of asthma and allergy in their control population was lower than expected.

A large unselected retrospective cohort study in Tennessee recently reported findings in support of a causal role for RSV bronchiolitis in asthma inception. In this study, Wu and colleagues[17] reported that children born 120 days before the peak of the RSV season had the greatest risk of hospitalization for lower respiratory tract illness and of asthma between 4 and 5.5 years of age.

However, several studies argue against a causal role for RSV in asthma inception. A large twin registry in Denmark was used to assess the relationships between severe

RSV illness and asthma development.[18,19] The data from this study suggest that severe RSV illnesses and asthma share a common predisposition, and although RSV can lead to short-term recurrent wheeze, it is not causal in long-term asthma development. Similarly, although the TCRS identified RSV wheezing illnesses during the first 3 years of life as an independent risk factor of wheezing at age 6 years, this relationship weakened over time and was no longer significant by age 13 years.[3] Thus, early RSV wheeze may lead to a recurrent wheeze phenotype, but it is less commonly associated with lifelong asthma. It would be interesting to determine whether the relationships reported from the Tennessee population-based study between 4 and 5.5 years of age persist over time.

The Role of HRV in Asthma

Recently, molecular diagnostics have allowed several groups to demonstrate that wheezing illnesses caused by HRV are potentially a more robust predictor of asthma development than episodes caused by RSV. Kotaniemi and colleagues[5] reported that children who were hospitalized with HRV wheezing illnesses during the first 2 years of life were at approximately fourfold increased risk of childhood asthma when compared with children hospitalized with wheezing associated with other viruses.

Two birth cohort studies have recently identified outpatient HRV wheezing illnesses as important predictors of childhood asthma development as well. The Childhood Origins of ASThma (COAST) study, a high-risk birth cohort examining the role of respiratory viruses and immune dysregulation in the development of asthma and other allergic diseases,[20] identified HRV wheezing illnesses during the first year of life as significant predictors of wheezing in the third year of life[21] and asthma at age 6 years.[6] In a similar high-risk birth cohort in Australia, Kusel and colleagues[22] reported that HRV wheezing illnesses during the first year of life were associated with increased asthma risk at age 5 years, although this finding was restricted to children who developed aeroallergen sensitization by age 2 years. In the COAST study, although HRV wheezing illnesses during infancy were an independent predictor of asthma development, children who wheezed with HRV and had aeroallergen sensitization during infancy had the greatest risk of asthma at school age.[6]

Age of Wheezing and Subsequent Asthma Risk

The COAST study has continued to evaluate specific viral cause and timing of wheezing illnesses as the children have progressed through early childhood. It seems that the age at which HRV wheezing illnesses occur has significant prognostic value with regard to subsequent asthma risk (Table 1). Children who wheezed with HRV during the first year of life had about a threefold risk of having asthma at age 6 years. HRV wheezing during the second year of life was associated with a more pronounced, about a sevenfold, increase in asthma risk, whereas wheezing with HRV infection during the third year of life was associated with a dramatic (odds ratio about 32) increase in asthma at school age. Nearly 90% of children who wheezed with HRV during the third year of life had asthma when they reached school age.[6] Long-term follow-up of these children to determine whether these relationships persist into the teenage years and beyond would prove very informative.

PROGRESSION FROM VIRUS-INDUCED WHEEZING TO ASTHMA

Preschool children with virus-induced wheezing use a disproportionate amount of health care resources compared with older children and adults with asthma,[1] in part because they do not respond as well to conventional asthma therapies. This, no

Table 1
Rhinovirus and RSV wheezing illnesses in years 1, 2, and 3, and risk of asthma at age 6 years

	Wheezing Illness	n	Asthma Age 6 Years (n)	Asthma Age 6 Years (%)	OR	95% CI	P Value
First year of life							
RSV	No	211	55	26	1.0		
	Yes	48	18	38	1.7	(0.9, 3.3)	0.11
RV	No	214	52	24	1.0		
	Yes	45	21	47	2.7	(1.4,5.3)	0.003
RV and RSV	Neither	192	46	24	1.0		
	RSV only	22	6	27	1.2	(0.4, 3.2)	0.73
	RV only	19	9	47	2.9	(1.1, 7.5)	0.03
	Both	26	12	46	2.7	(1.2, 6.3)	0.02
Second year of life							
RSV	No	231	61	26	1.0		
	Yes	28	12	43	2.1	(0.9, 4.7)	0.07
RV	No	222	49	22	1.0		
	Yes	37	24	65	6.5	(3.1, 13.7)	<0.0001
RV and RSV	Neither	203	44	22	1.0		
	RSV only	19	5	26	1.3	(0.4, 3.8)	0.64
	RV only	28	17	61	5.6	(2.4, 12.8)	<0.000l
	Both	9	7	78	12.6	(2.5, 63.1)	0.002
Third year of life							
RSV	No	242	60	25	1.0		
	Yes	17	13	76	9.9	(3.1, 31.4)	0.0001
RV	No	225	43	19	1.0		
	Yes	34	30	88	31.7	(10.6, 94.9)	<0.0001
RV and RSV	Neither	214	35	16	1.0		
	RSV only	11	8	73	13.6	(3.4, 54.0)	0.0002
	RV only	28	25	89	42.6	(12.2, 148.9)	<0.0001
	Both	6	5	83	25.6	(2.9, 225.6)	0.004

Abbreviations: CI, confidence interval; OR, odds ratio; RV, rhinovirus.

Data From Jackson DJ, Gangnon RE, Evans MD, et al. Wheezing rhinovirus illnesses in early life predict asthma development in high-risk children. Am J Respir Crit Care Med 2008; 178(7):667–72.

doubt, is also due to the heterogeneity of this population, including children who outgrow their wheezing and those who continue to wheeze into school age and beyond.

In the Preventing Early Asthma in Kids study, a trial comparing treatment with low-dose fluticasone to placebo in high-risk children with recurrent wheezing, it was observed that for children who did not outgrow their wheezing, lower respiratory symptom burden progressively increased as they advanced through the preschool years.[23] Multiple cohort studies have demonstrated that there are long-lasting effects on lung function for children who begin wheezing before age 3 years and develop persistent disease. In the TCRS, children who began wheezing before age 3 years and continued to wheeze at school age had reductions in lung function at age 6 years[2] that persisted at least to the teenage years.[24] Illi and colleagues,[25] through careful assessment of allergic sensitization and exposure, demonstrated that children who wheezed during the preschool years, were sensitized to aeroallergens, and continued to wheeze had impairment in lung function to at least age 13 years.

However, partly because of the invasive nature of the procedures necessary to directly study the lower airway, there is a paucity of data to help us understand the underlying pathogenesis of loss of lung function in children who start with recurrent virus-induced wheezing but develop persistent disease. Nonetheless, a few studies may shed some light on the inflammatory processes that occur in these children. Krawiec and colleagues[26] performed bronchoscopy and bronchoalveolar lavage on children of median age 15 months with recurrent wheezing and to a group of healthy controls. These studies demonstrated that children with persistent wheezing had increased inflammatory cells and markers of inflammation compared with healthy controls but did not have the characteristic eosinophil predominance seen in older children and adults with asthma. Similarly, Saglani and colleagues[27] performed bronchoscopy and biopsy in children of median age 12 months with persistent wheezing and were unable to demonstrate either eosinophilic inflammation or reticular basement membrane (RBM) thickening, both common features of asthma seen in older children and adults. In contrast, in further studies of older children with recurrent wheezing of median age 29 months, they were able to demonstrate the presence of eosinophilic inflammation and RBM thickening when compared with a group of controls. This suggests that inflammatory changes and remodeling typical of asthma develop between 1 and 3 years of age in recurrently wheezing children and highlights the potential importance of environmental exposures, such as virus infections, during this period.

MECHANISMS BY WHICH VIRUSES MAY PROMOTE ASTHMA INCEPTION

Several animal models have suggested mechanisms by which virus infection in early life could cause asthma inception. The COAST study was based on a rat model of virus-induced airway dysfunction in which a histologic and physiologic asthma phenotype could be induced only in a genetically predisposed Th2-biased strain when they were infected at a critical time in the development of the lung and/or the immune system (weanling ago).[28] However, there is limited data in humans demonstrating distinct mechanisms for causality of virus infections in asthma inception. Several recent human studies suggest plausible mechanisms by which HRV could be involved in airway remodeling and asthma inception.

Leigh and colleagues[29] demonstrated that in vitro infection of airway epithelial cells with HRV led to increased production of several mediators involved in airway remodeling, including amphiregulin, activin A, and vascular endothelial growth factor (VEGF). The authors also found increased VEGF in nasal lavage fluid of volunteers with natural HRV infections. In another epithelial cell model, Zhu and colleagues[30] found that HRV infection led to toll-like receptor 3-dependent mucin production and upregulation of epidermal growth factor receptor, a prominent component of epithelial repair. Finally, epithelial cell gene expression studies have identified several potential novel pathways involved in the response to HRV infection. Proud and colleagues[31] found that HRV infection led to upregulation of many genes, perhaps most notably in interferon and airway repair and remodeling pathways. Bochkov and colleagues[32] similarly demonstrated that HRV infection led to upregulation of a number of genes involved in interferon and airway remodeling pathways. In this study, differences between asthmatics and controls were similar before and during HRV infection. In summary, although data that demonstrates causality of HRV infection in asthma inception are limited, several plausible mechanisms by which recurrent HRV infection could lead to airway damage and remodeling have been identified and are deserving of further study.

HOST FACTORS ASSOCIATED WITH WHEEZING AND ASTHMA

If viruses are causal in asthma inception, this is likely to be particularly true in susceptible hosts (**Fig. 1**). A so-called two-hit hypothesis has been proposed,[20] whereby children with immune dysregulation (favoring an allergic phenotype) who develop a lower respiratory viral illness during a critical time in development progress to an asthma phenotype. Allergic sensitization during early childhood has been identified by several studies as an important risk factor of asthma development.[6,22,25] In older children with asthma, allergic sensitization is a risk factor of more severe upper and lower respiratory viral illnesses.[33,34] Several observations may help explain host susceptibility to virus-induced wheezing and asthma exacerbations.

Interferons are known to play an important role in the host response to virus infections, and there is growing data to support a prominent role for interferons in the pathogenesis of virus-induced wheezing and asthma. Gern and colleagues[35] linked

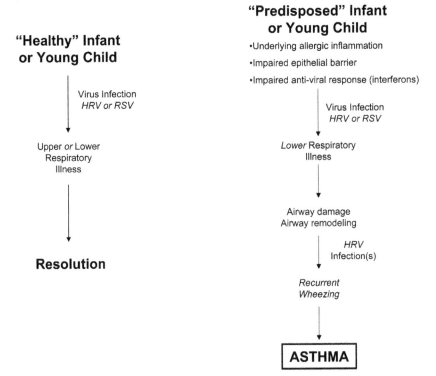

Fig. 1. The potential consequences of virus infections in young children and how recurrent virus infection, particularly with HRV, may be causal in asthma pathogenesis in predisposed children.

immature peripheral blood interferon-γ responses to mitogens and viruses at birth with recurrent wheezing during infancy. Similarly, Stern and colleagues[36] connected reduced peripheral blood interferon-γ responses to mitogen at 9 months of age to an increased risk of wheezing in toddlers and school-aged children. Peripheral blood mononuclear cells from adult asthmatics produce less interferon-γ in response to HRV infection than controls,[37] and the degree of impairment correlates with airway hyper-responsiveness and degree of airway obstruction.[38]

Several other investigators, through experiments on airway epithelial cells and in peripheral blood, have identified deficiencies in interferons as an important potential mechanism for asthmatics' susceptibility to more severe HRV illnesses. Wark and colleagues.[39] demonstrated that bronchial epithelial cells from atopic asthmatics infected with HRV in vitro have deficient interferon-β (a type I interferon) responses when compared with controls. In this study, the decreased interferon-β response was associated with delayed apoptosis and increased viral replication, which was overcome with the addition of exogenous interferon-β. Additionally, lower levels of interferon-α (another type I interferon) responses have been demonstrated in the peripheral blood of children[40] and adults[41] with atopic asthma versus nonatopic controls. Finally, Contoli and colleagues[42] found that bronchial epithelial cells and alveolar macrophages from atopic asthmatics had impaired interferon-λ (a type III interferon) responses to HRV infection and that these responses correlated with decline of forced expiratory volume in the first second of expiration during exacerbations. Although these studies have identified defects in interferon pathways as potential important contributors to early childhood wheezing and asthma, unfortunately, attempts to replicate these findings have not always been successful. Two recent studies found no difference in epithelial cell responses between asthmatics and controls.[32,43]

Another important component of the innate immune response to virus infection is barrier function. Barrier function of the skin is important in the pathogenesis of atopic dermatitis, with filaggrin mutations identified in several patients with severe atopic dermatitis.[44] Ongoing allergic inflammation may lead to a local or acquired filaggrin deficit.[45] Several studies have highlighted how disruption of the airway epithelium could alter host antiviral responses and severity of lower respiratory illnesses. In fact, filaggrin mutations have been identified as a risk factor of asthma and asthma exacerbations in children.[46,47] A unique model of airway injury took this observation one step further in demonstrating the potential consequences of impairment in airway barrier function through physical injury. Jakiela and colleagues,[48] using in vitro epithelial cell culture, showed that mechanical injury to the epithelia resulted in increased replication of HRV. This is a potential mechanism by which various host factors or environmental exposures, such as allergen, tobacco smoke, and previous virus infection, could lead to impairment in barrier function, increased viral replication, and more severe lower respiratory illnesses.

SUMMARY

Respiratory viruses are a major cause of morbidity in young children. Wheezing illnesses caused by viruses during early life are the most common initial presentation of childhood asthma. Recent evidence suggests that wheezing with HRV is the most robust predictor of subsequent asthma. However, whether HRV is causal in asthma inception is an open question. Plausible mechanisms of causality have been identified but are in need of further study. The most definitive way to prove causality would be to prevent HRV infection and demonstrate reductions in asthma development, but vaccines for HRV have proven elusive, in part due to the nearly 150 existing species of HRV. Studies attempting to identify more virulent or asthmogenic forms of HRV are ongoing and could prove very informative. Novel preventive and therapeutic strategies are sorely needed to prevent or interrupt the progression from virus-induced wheezing to persistent asthma.

REFERENCES

1. Akinbami LJ, Moorman JE, Garbe PL, et al. Status of childhood asthma in the United States, 1980–2007. Pediatrics 2009;123(Suppl 3):S131–45.
2. Martinez FD, Wright AL, Taussig LM, et al. Asthma and wheezing in the first six years of life. N Engl J Med 1995;332:133–8.
3. Stein RT, Sherrill D, Morgan WJ, et al. Respiratory syncytial virus in early life and risk of wheeze and allergy by age 13 years. Lancet 1999;354:541–5.
4. Sigurs N, Gustafsson PM, Bjarnason R, et al. Severe respiratory syncytial virus bronchiolitis in infancy and asthma and allergy at age 13. Am J Respir Crit Care Med 2005;171(2):137–41.
5. Kotaniemi-Syrjanen A, Vainionpaa R, Reijonen TM, et al. Rhinovirus-induced wheezing in infancy–the first sign of childhood asthma? J Allergy Clin Immunol 2003;111(1):66–71.
6. Jackson DJ, Gangnon RE, Evans MD, et al. Wheezing rhinovirus illnesses in early life predict asthma development in high-risk children. Am J Respir Crit Care Med 2008;178(7):667–72.
7. Taussig LM, Wright AL, Holberg CJ, et al. Tucson children's respiratory study: 1980 to present. J Allergy Clin Immunol 2003;111(4):661–75.
8. Openshaw PJM. Immunological mechanisms in respiratory syncytial virus disease. Springer Semin Immunopathol 1995;17:187–201.
9. Simoes EA. Environmental and demographic risk factors for respiratory syncytial virus lower respiratory tract disease. J Pediatr 2003;143(Suppl 5):S118–26.
10. Miller EK, Lu X, Erdman DD, et al. Rhinovirus-associated hospitalizations in young children. J Infect Dis 2007;195(6):773–81.
11. Jartti T, Lehtinen P, Vuorinen T, et al. Bronchiolitis: age and previous wheezing episodes are linked to viral etiology and atopic characteristics. Pediatr Infect Dis J 2009;28(4):311–7.
12. Lee WM, Kiesner C, Pappas T, et al. A diverse group of previously unrecognized human rhinoviruses are common causes of respiratory illnesses in infants. PLoS One 2007;2(10):e966.
13. Miller EK, Edwards KM, Weinberg GA, et al. A novel group of rhinoviruses is associated with asthma hospitalizations. J Allergy Clin Immunol 2009;123(1):98–104.
14. Miller EK, Khuri-Bulos N, Williams JV, et al. Human rhinovirus C associated with wheezing in hospitalised children in the Middle East. J Clin Virol 2009;46(1):85–9.
15. Tan BH, Loo LH, Lim EA, et al. Human rhinovirus group C in hospitalized children, Singapore. Emerg Infect Dis 2009;15(8):1318–20.
16. McErlean P, Shackelton LA, Andrews E, et al. Distinguishing molecular features and clinical characteristics of a putative new rhinovirus species, human rhinovirus C (HRV C). PLoS One 2008;3(4):e1847.
17. Wu P, Dupont WD, Griffin MR, et al. Evidence of a causal role of winter virus infection during infancy in early childhood asthma. Am J Respir Crit Care Med 2008; 178(11):1123–9.
18. Thomsen SF, van der SS, Stensballe LG, et al. Exploring the association between severe respiratory syncytial virus infection and asthma: a registry-based twin study. Am J Respir Crit Care Med 2009;179(12):1091–7.

19. Stensballe LG, Simonsen JB, Thomsen SF, et al. The causal direction in the association between respiratory syncytial virus hospitalization and asthma. J Allergy Clin Immunol 2009;123(1):131–7.

20. Lemanske RF Jr. The childhood origins of asthma (COAST) study. Pediatr Allergy Immunol 2002;13(Suppl):1538–43.

21. Lemanske RF Jr, Jackson DJ, Gangnon RE, et al. Rhinovirus illnesses during infancy predict subsequent childhood wheezing. J Allergy Clin Immunol 2005;116(3):571–7.

22. Kusel MM, de Klerk NH, Kebadze T, et al. Early-life respiratory viral infections, atopic sensitization, and risk of subsequent development of persistent asthma. J Allergy Clin Immunol 2007;119(5):1105–10.

23. Guilbert TW, Morgan WJ, Zeiger RS, et al. Long-term inhaled corticosteroids in preschool children at high risk for asthma. N Engl J Med 2006;354(19):1985–97.

24. Morgan WJ, Stern DA, Sherrill DL, et al. Outcome of asthma and wheezing in the first 6 years of life: follow-up through adolescence. Am J Respir Crit Care Med 2005;172(10):1253–8.

25. Illi S, von Mutius E, Lau S, et al. Perennial allergen sensitisation early in life and chronic asthma in children: a birth cohort study. Lancet 2006;368(9537):763–70.

26. Krawiec ME, Westcott JY, Chu HW, et al. Persistent wheezing in very young children is associated with lower respiratory inflammation. Am J Respir Crit Care Med 2001;163(6):1338–43.

27. Saglani S, Malmstrom K, Pelkonen AS, et al. Airway remodeling and inflammation in symptomatic infants with reversible airflow obstruction. Am J Respir Crit Care Med 2005;171(7):722–7.

28. Rosenthal LA, Amineva SP, Szakaly RJ, et al. A rat model of picornavirus-induced airway infection and inflammation. Virol J 2009;6:122.

29. Leigh R, Oyelusi W, Wiehler S, et al. Human rhinovirus infection enhances airway epithelial cell production of growth factors involved in airway remodeling. J Allergy Clin Immunol 2008;121(5):1238–45.

30. Zhu L, Lee PK, Lee WM, et al. Rhinovirus-induced major airway mucin production involves a novel TLR3-EGFR-dependent pathway. Am J Respir Cell Mol Biol 2009; 40(5):610–9.

31. Proud D, Turner RB, Winther B, et al. Gene expression profiles during in vivo human rhinovirus infection: insights into the host response. Am J Respir Crit Care Med 2008;178(9):962–8.

32. Bochkov YA, Hanson KM, Keles S, et al. Rhinovirus-induced modulation of gene expression in bronchial epithelial cells from subjects with asthma. Mucosal Immunol 2009;3(1):69–80.

33. Olenec JP, Kim WK, Lee WM, et al. Weekly monitoring of children with asthma for infections and illness during common cold seasons. J Allergy Clin Immunol 2010; 125(5):1001–6.

34. Heymann PW, Carper HT, Murphy DD, et al. Viral infections in relation to age, atopy, and season of admission among children hospitalized for wheezing. J Allergy Clin Immunol 2004;114(2):239–47.

35. Gern JE, Brooks GD, Meyer P, et al. Bidirectional interactions between viral respiratory illnesses and cytokine responses in the first year of life. J Allergy Clin Immunol 2006;117(1):72–8.

36. Stern DA, Guerra S, Halonen M, et al. Low IFN-gamma production in the first year of life as a predictor of wheeze during childhood. J Allergy Clin Immunol 2007; 120(4):835–41.

37. Papadopoulos NG, Stanciu LA, Papi A, et al. A defective type 1 response to rhinovirus in atopic asthma. Thorax 2002;57(4):328–32.

38. Brooks GD, Buchta KA, Swenson CA, et al. Rhinovirus-induced interferon-gamma and airway responsiveness in asthma. Am J Respir Crit Care Med 2003;168(9):1091–4.
39. Wark PA, Johnston SL, Bucchieri F, et al. Asthmatic bronchial epithelial cells have a deficient innate immune response to infection with rhinovirus. J Exp Med 2005; 201(6):937–47.
40. Bufe A, Gehlhar K, Grage-Griebenow E, et al. Atopic phenotype in children is associated with decreased virus-induced interferon-alpha release. Int Arch Allergy Immunol 2002;127(1):82–8.
41. Gehlhar K, Bilitewski C, Reinitz-Rademacher K, et al. Impaired virus-induced interferon-alpha2 release in adult asthmatic patients. Clin Exp Allergy 2006; 36(3):331–7.
42. Contoli M, Message SD, Laza-Stanca V, et al. Role of deficient type III interferon-lambda production in asthma exacerbations. Nat Med 2006;12:1023–6.
43. Lopez-Souza N, Favoreto S, Wong H, et al. In vitro susceptibility to rhinovirus infection is greater for bronchial than for nasal airway epithelial cells in human subjects. J Allergy Clin Immunol 2009;123(6):1384–90.
44. Palmer CN, Irvine AD, Terron-Kwiatkowski A, et al. Common loss-of-function variants of the epidermal barrier protein filaggrin are a major predisposing factor for atopic dermatitis. Nat Genet 2006;38(4):441–6.
45. Howell MD, Kim BE, Gao P, et al. Cytokine modulation of atopic dermatitis filaggrin skin expression. J Allergy Clin Immunol 2007;120(1):150–5.
46. Basu K, Palmer CN, Lipworth BJ, et al. Filaggrin null mutations are associated with increased asthma exacerbations in children and young adults. Allergy 2008;63(9):1211–7.
47. McLean WH, Palmer CN, Henderson J, et al. Filaggrin variants confer susceptibility to asthma. J Allergy Clin Immunol 2008;121(5):1294–5.
48. Jakiela B, Brockman-Schneider R, Amineva S, et al. Basal cells of differentiated bronchial epithelium are more susceptible to rhinovirus infection. Am J Respir Cell Mol Biol 2008;38(5):517–23.

Respiratory Syncytial Virus Infections in the Adult Asthmatic – Mechanisms of Host Susceptibility and Viral Subversion

Blair D. Westerly, MD[a], R. Stokes Peebles Jr, MD[b],*

KEYWORDS

• Respiratory syncytial virus • Asthma • Wheezing • Adults

Respiratory syncytial virus (RSV), a single-stranded RNA virus of the Paramyxoviri-dae family, is a major cause of bronchiolitis in infants and is also conjectured to be an early-life influence on the development of asthma.[1,2] Although the data supporting a role for RSV in bronchiolitis in children are robust and evidence to support its role in juvenile asthmatics exists, RSV's role in asthma pathogenesis in adults is not as clearly defined. The authors review the literature to further elucidate RSV's impact on adult asthmatics, including its importance as a cause of asthma exacerbations. They examine the morbidity associated with RSV infection and how the immune response may differ between adult asthmatics and nonasthmatics. They review the responses by specific cell types from adults with asthma that are stimulated by RSV. They also consider the role of early-life exposure to RSV and its contribution to asthma in adults. Lastly, they review the mechanisms by which RSV evades normal host immune responses and subverts these responses to its benefit.

This work was supported by R01-HL-090664, R01-AI070672, and 1I01BX000624.
The authors declare no conflict of interest.
[a] Department of Medicine, Vanderbilt University School of Medicine, Vanderbilt University Medical Center, 1161 21st Avenue South, Nashville, TN 37232, USA
[b] Division of Allergy, Pulmonary, and Critical Care Medicine, Department of Medicine, Vanderbilt University School of Medicine, Vanderbilt University Medical Center, 1161 21st Avenue South, Nashville, TN 37232, USA
* Corresponding author. T-1217 MCN, Vanderbilt University Medical Center, Nashville, TN 37232-2650.
E-mail address: stokes.peebles@vanderbilt.edu

RSV IN ADULTS AND ITS IMPACT ON ASTHMA EXACERBATIONS
How Important is RSV as a Cause of Asthma Exacerbations?

Although not as settled as the data supporting RSV as a cause of bronchiolitis in young children, evidence also supports RSV as an important cause of acute respiratory illness in adults. Compared with healthy adults, patients who are at high risk of complications of respiratory illness, including those with asthma, are more likely to require hospitalization when infected with RSV.[3] In a prospective study of subjects aged 15 to 56 years with atopic asthma who recorded symptom scores and daily peak flow rates, viruses were detected in approximately 60% of asthma exacerbations that were associated with symptoms of a respiratory tract infection, with RSV being the most common virus detected.[4] In this same study, roughly 60% of children with allergic asthma had symptoms of a respiratory infection associated with an asthma exacerbation, and RSV was also the most commonly detected virus in this age group.[4] Viral assays based on the polymerase chain reaction (PCR) were not available at that time for viral detection, and therefore the true incidence of viral cause may have been skewed by the limited diagnostic methods available, because only about 30% of those with exacerbations had detectable virus.

In a prospective study of hospitalized patients over a 4-year period to determine the frequency of specific viral infections that caused respiratory illness severe enough to require hospitalization in patients with chronic illness, RSV was the most commonly detected virus. In this study, 80% of the infections leading to hospitalization were in children younger than 5 years, whereas RSV was detected in 17% of adults hospitalized for respiratory symptoms.[5] One of the caveats of studying the epidemiology of RSV and its contribution to respiratory diseases, such as asthma, is that this virus has a narrow seasonality; therefore, if a study is performed in the summer, RSV may be underrepresented, and if performed in the winter, RSV could possibly be overrepresented as a cause of respiratory infection when compared with other viruses. Therefore, the season in which the study is performed is crucial in accounting for these potential limitations. Because the investigators collected data for 4 entire years, the potential bias of RSV's seasonality was reduced in this study.[5]

Even with some evidence supporting the role of RSV in adult asthma exacerbations, other studies have not as clearly implicated RSV. In a study of adult controls and asthmatics without symptoms of an acute exacerbation, sputum was induced with 3% sodium chloride solution and oropharyngeal specimens were analyzed by PCR or reverse transcriptase (RT)-PCR to assess the role of different bacteria and viruses in stable asthma.[6] In this study, positivity for rhinovirus, *Chlamydophila pneumoniae* or *Bordetella pertussis*, was associated with significant reductions in forced expiratory volume in 1 second (FEV_1), FEV_1/forced vital capacity (FVC), or symptoms, but RSV was not.[6]

In a prospective study of 79 adult asthmatics with exacerbations requiring hospitalization over a 12-month period, 37% of exacerbations were thought to have infectious cause, but only one of the 24 confirmed viral infections implicated RSV.[7] This study used serologic testing and cultures of nasopharyngeal aspirates for detection of virus or bacteria, which may have resulted in lower sensitivity for detecting infections than more sensitive diagnostic tests, such as PCR. Retrospectively, other early studies attempting to define the role of viruses in asthma exacerbations seem to have been limited by the technology available for viral detection.[8,9] One study analyzed the incidence of acute asthma and bronchitis over an 11-year period; it was able to demonstrate increased asthma rates and exacerbations with increasing circulating virus levels based on epidemiologic viral isolation data but could not causally implicate RSV or any other virus specifically.[10]

A longitudinal study of adult asthmatics over a 22-month period examined symptomatic colds and asthma exacerbations; it confirmed RSV positivity only once in the 119 documented upper respiratory tract infections and only once in the 27 infections associated with an objective exacerbation, diagnosed by symptoms and decrease in peak flow.[8] This study used serum serologic conversion for detection of most respiratory viruses, including RSV, but used PCR for human rhinovirus, the most commonly detected virus. PCR testing for RSV and many other viruses was not yet available at the time of the study, and lack of diagnostic sensitivity probably accounted for the low recognized contribution of these viruses.

Another smaller prospective study, which attempted to delineate the role of viral infections in exacerbations of adult asthmatics, used rapid antigen detection and viral culture in all patients presenting to the emergency department with symptoms of an exacerbation over a 7-month period during fall and winter.[9] Even with the addition of serum antibody titers in about half the patients, this study found no positivity for RSV in the population, and furthermore, no positivity for many other common respiratory viruses was found, including influenza A or B, parainfluenza 1, 2 or 3, adenovirus, or rhinovirus.[9] The investigators concluded that there may be an overstated importance of respiratory viruses in asthma exacerbations, but the lack of PCR use calls into question that specific conclusion. Furthermore, it has been shown that viral exacerbation causes have varied with subject age and diagnostic methods used for viral detection,[11] with adults producing less respiratory secretions than children, further complicating diagnosis in adults.[8,12]

MORBIDITY ASSOCIATED WITH RSV INFECTIONS

RSV is an important cause of morbidity in adults and can result in hospitalization and resource use, especially during winter when the incidence of viral infections increases.[3,5,13–18] In a study conducted over 3 years in the United Kingdom, from 10% to 22% of patients who visited a physician for a winter respiratory illness had an RSV infection detected by RT-PCR.[19] In a prospective viral surveillance study over 20 years during the months in which RSV is known to be active in the community, 7% of adults had RSV infection, of which 84% (177/211) were symptomatic.[16] In a retrospective study of a 10-year period in Ontario, Canada designed to study seasonal and temporal patterns of primary-care visits for respiratory illnesses, RSV was demonstrated to have a significant influence on visits related to asthma, chronic obstructive pulmonary disease (COPD), and pneumonia, as well as a seasonal influence on the use of health services, with winter visits threefold higher than summer visits.[17] Furthermore, a retrospective analysis of the viral cause of patients hospitalized for respiratory illness found that among patients with chronic pulmonary disease, RSV accounted for 10.4% of such hospitalizations and, together with influenza and parainfluenza, was responsible for 75% of all viral infections requiring hospitalization.[5]

In a prospective surveillance study over 4 consecutive winters, another group evaluated morbidity associated with RSV in healthy adults older than 65 years and adults with chronic heart or lung disease and found that RSV disease burden was similar to that of influenza (3%–7% in healthy adults and 4%–10% in high-risk adults).[3] Furthermore, RSV accounted for 10.6% of hospital admissions for pneumonia, 11.4% of admissions for COPD, 5.4% of congestive heart failure (CHF) admissions, and 7.2% of asthma admissions.[3] The use of health-care services related to RSV infection was similar to that of influenza among high risk adults, and RSV-related hospitalizations are estimated to cost more than $1 billion annually.[3,14] A retrospective cohort study of patients with chronic lung disease showed RSV to be implicated in 18 per 1000 hospitalizations and 5 per 1000 deaths in the elderly each year.[15] The mortality associated with RSV in this large study was 46 per 10,000 persons in those older than 65 years with chronic lung disease and 15.3 per 10,000 in subjects aged 50 to 64 years.[15] Another estimate using viral surveillance and national databases proposed that RSV was responsible for about 10,000 deaths annually in the United States in those older than 65 years.[18] Moreover, treatment of RSV and influenza accounted for 12% to 14% of antibiotic use in adults with chronic lung disease.[15] RSV-infected patients have been shown to have physical examination findings (wheezing and rhonchi) and laboratory findings (no leukocytosis) that may distinguish RSV infections from bacterial infections[13]; not considering RSV in the differential diagnosis for such patients is a major hindrance to making the diagnosis.

RSV may also be important as a potential nosocomial infection, especially in hospitalized patients already suffering from respiratory disease or respiratory failure. In a small cohort of intubated patients over a 2-month period, 5 of the 11 adult patients on mechanical ventilation in the medical intensive care unit (mean age 47.8+/−15.0 years) had evidence of RSV infection, and the mortality rate in this population was 40%.[20] Analysis of adults admitted to the hospital during the winter of 2007 to 2008 who had RSV infection identified by quantitative RT-PCR revealed significantly higher nasal viral loads in patients requiring mechanical ventilation than in nonventilated patients, and these higher viral loads were independently associated with respiratory failure.[21] In this same study, significantly more patients hospitalized with RSV had cardiopulmonary disease and COPD, and there was a trend toward asthma as well ($P = .06$); but the study was underpowered for this endpoint.[21] Therefore, with the advent of more sensitive assays to detect specific viruses, the importance of RSV as a cause of significant morbidity in adults has become more apparent.

IMMUNE RESPONSE TO RSV INFECTION IN NONASTHMATIC ADULTS

The immune response by humans to RSV infection consists of humoral and cellular components and related cytokine signaling, with an intricate interaction among cell types from both arms of the immune response. After initial stimulation of dendritic cells in the nasal mucosa[22,23] in similar fashion to other viruses, it is generally thought that humoral responses, serum and secretory, are important for protection from RSV infection, whereas cellular immunity is probably the most important for viral clearance. However, given that recurrent RSV infection is the rule throughout an individual's life, immunity seems incomplete.

Humoral Immunity in Host Defense

Many studies have examined the role of humoral immunity in host defense to RSV, including which viral proteins serve as antigens recognized for sustained immunity. Early in the study of host immune responses to RSV in children, recurrent disease was noted to be common, and multiple infections were needed before a sustained response could be detected serologically.[24] Nonmaternal antibodies could only be discerned after age 3 months; however, no antibody to the surface glycoprotein was detected in children younger than 1 year.[25] A broadening of the antibody response occurred with increasing age, including a response to the surface fusion protein (F protein) in IgM and IgA classes, but only rarely was an inclusive response found to all viral proteins.[25] Furthermore, the initial antibody response in Kenyan infants has been shown to be RSV genotype-specific to the variable region of the RSV G protein, with cross-reactivity developing with subsequent infections.[26] In healthy adults, those with lower serum neutralizing antibodies and serum IgG titers to F protein were at higher risk of infection after inoculation with live RSV.[27] For RSV challenge in young healthy adults, nasal neutralizing IgA correlated more with protection than serum neutralizing antibodies.[28] The protective effect of humoral immunity demonstrated in this challenge study has also been duplicated in community dwellers.[29] Those naturally infected with RSV had lower RSV-specific nasal IgA, serum IgG to F, G_A, and G_B, and neutralizing antibodies to group A and B strains, and multivariate analysis demonstrated that lower serum IgG and nasal IgA levels were independent risk factors of infection.[29] In healthy volunteers, RSV neutralizing antibodies to F or G_A protein were protective, but up to a quarter of the subjects were re-infected regardless of antibody titers, and by 8 months after initial inoculation, almost two-thirds could be re-infected.[30] In another study, adults infected with RSV showed a mean eightfold increase in antibody titers, but at 1 year, 75% had at least a fourfold drop in these titers.[26]

Given that RSV infection tends to be most severe in the elderly, the effect of age on antibody production and protection has been examined in multiple studies.[31,32] In one study, older patients had higher mean antibody titers than their younger counterparts at baseline but did not have increased neutralizing activity.[31] Of those elderly and young patients infected naturally with RSV during the study, no difference was seen in the immune response, with 79% of older subjects achieving a fourfold increase or greater in microneutralization assay titers to RSV antigens F, G_A, and G_B, whereas only 64% of young subjects had a similar increase.[31] The investigators hypothesized that a recent RSV infection may be responsible for the oldest, frailest subjects in the study having the highest antibody titers, especially given the high rate of acute respiratory illnesses seen in adult day-care centers,[33] or that the humoral dysregulation or dysfunction that accompanies increasing age may be at play.

In a separate study, although antibody levels were similar in young and old adults at baseline, older individuals had significantly greater neutralizing antibody production to both strains of RSV and increased responses to specific RSV antigens F, G_A, and G_B.[32] In this study, there was a trend toward higher viral titers in seroresponders compared with nonresponders, but the investigators also speculated that the boosted humoral response might be a reflection of a shift from a Th1- to a Th2-subtype response, given the evidence of diminished T-cell responses to RSV in aged mouse models and older persons.[34–37] Furthermore, the ratio of neutralizing antibodies pre- and postinoculation were similar between the 2 groups, suggesting a similar qualitative response in the young and the old.[32] Although 85% of elderly nursing home residents with positive RSV culture had a greater than fourfold increase in RSV-specific IgG, acute antibody titers were similar to those residents without RSV infection. There was no correlation between antibody titers and severity of illness, causing the investigators to question the protective effect of antibodies in acquiring the illness or modulating its severity.[38] Another study did show low serum-neutralizing antibody titers to be a significant risk factor of increased severity of disease in healthy elderly adults and high-risk young adults (odds ratio = 5.89).[39] Furthermore, a later study found that serum neutralizing antibodies were much more likely to be found in younger patients than in frail patients (92.00% vs 36.21%) at baseline.[40] Therefore, the discrepancy in the results suggests that there are factors other than age that regulate humoral responses to RSV.

Cellular Immunity

Although the effectiveness of humoral immunity for protection from RSV infection may still be debatable, cellular immunity plays a role in clearance of RSV-infected cells.[41] The role of cytotoxic T cells (MHC class I-restricted) was examined in RSV-infected adults and it was shown that nine of the 10 viral proteins were recognized by cytotoxic

T cells when B lymphoblastoid cells were infected with recombinant vaccinia viruses with genes for single RSV proteins, of which the nucleoprotein N and surface proteins SH and F were most strongly recognized.[42] The G protein, an antigen commonly evaluated for the humoral immune response, was rarely recognized (2/9).[42] Others have attempted to elucidate the balance between proinflammatory cells (CD4, Th1, and CD8) and anti-inflammatory cells (CD4, Th2) in RSV infection, by measuring cytokines associated with specific cell types in healthy elderly and healthy young adults.[43] To this end, elderly subjects had a decreased interleukin (IL)-10/interferon (IFN)-γ ratio (CD4 cells only) compared with young adults, indicating, perhaps, a predominance of proinflammatory T cells in the elderly that might account for the more severe clinical syndrome seen in this population.[43] There was no difference in the number of IL-10- or IFN-γ-producing cells between young and old, but RSV-induced IFN-γ responses were stronger for CD4 cells than CD8 cells, leading the investigators to speculate that increased disease severity in the elderly may be related to the older subjects' inability to rapidly expand CD8 replication in the setting of infection.[43,44] In fact, one study was able to show that memory T-cell populations for RSV are lower for elderly patients and those with COPD, and they required in vitro expansion to detect RSV-specific CD8 memory cells.[45]

Cytokines and Virus Infection

Cytokines and other signaling molecules produced by immune cells during an RSV infection are a reflection of the cell types that predominate in clearing the virus. Just as nasal IgA has been demonstrated to have a protective effect against RSV infection,[28,29] cytokines and chemokines found in the nasal secretions of patients with RSV infection act as chemoattractants for the immune cells in response to the virus. Peripheral blood mononuclear cells (PBMCs) of adults and children previously infected with RSV showed an RSV-specific response with Th1-type cytokines, IFN-γ and IL-2, without similar responses in IL-4 or IL-5.[46] In healthy, nonsmoking adults inoculated with live RSV, there was increased IL-8 in nasal lavage specimens during and after infection, along with increased levels of regulated upon activation, normal T-cell expressed, and secreted (RANTES), macrophage inhibitory protein (MIP)-1α, and monocyte chemotactic protein (MCP)-1 at the time of viral shedding.[47] It has also been shown that through upregulation of toll-like receptor 3 and protein kinase R, RSV increases nuclear factor kappa-light-chain-enhancer of activated B cells (NF-κB), and thus, IL-8 production.[48]

As was seen with humoral and cellular immunity with RSV infection, the cytokine response differs in healthy populations between younger and older subjects. When cultured PBMCs were presented with RSV by autologous dendritic cells, older subjects' PBMCs produced significantly fewer IFN-γ enzyme-linked immunospots than younger subjects' PBMCs.[35] The authors suggest that this may be due to an aging defect in T-cell response to RSV as previously described,[34,36,49] especially in the face of using dendritic cells to maximize costimulation versus using PBMCs alone.[35]

Association of Host Cytokine Genotype with RSV-induced Immune Responses

Because of the influence of cytokines on the immune response and the severity of illness in viral respiratory infections, a few studies have been conducted to evaluate the potential impact of gene polymorphisms on cytokine responses to RSV in adults and children.[50,51] Using DNA extracted from adults experimentally inoculated with RSV, one group was able to genotype the cytokine response using PCR-sequence–specific primer technology.[51] They found that IFN-γ genotype could predict IL-1 levels, with low IFN-γ producers (genotype A/A) making more IL-1 and high IFN-γ producers (genotype T/T or T/A) making less IL-1; furthermore, they showed that tumor necrosis factor (TNF)-α genotype could predict IL-6 and IL-8 protein levels, again in an inverse fashion, with low TNF-α producers (genotype G/G) making more IL-6 and IL-8 than high TNF-α producers (genotype G/A or A/A).[51] Additionally, throat and general symptoms correlated with IL-6 protein levels but not with the IL-6 genotype.[44] A similar study in children hospitalized with confirmed RSV infection showed that IFN-γ genotypes could predict severity of lower respiratory illness (higher producers, genotype T/T or T/A, were more severe), duration of intensive care unit (ICU) stay (high producers, genotype T/T or T/A, stayed longer), and frequency of acute otitis media (low producers, genotype A/A, had more episodes), whereas the IL-6 genotype inversely correlated with length of oxygen supplementation and hospital stay, with high producers (genotype G/G or G/C) needing less oxygen and shorter stays than low producers (genotype C/C).[50] High production levels of IFN-γ had a protective effect on otitis media but detrimental effect on the severity of lower respiratory tract illness and duration of ICU stay, for which the authors speculated that it reflected the degree of infection localization. IL-10 (low producers, ACC/ACC, ACC/ATA, or ATA/ATA genotypes) and transforming growth factor (TGF)-β1 (C/C-G/C, C/C-C/C, T/T-C/C, or T/C-C/C genotypes) polymorphisms were predictive of likelihood of pneumonia and low oxygen saturations at presentation, respectively in infants, whereas these 2 cytokine genotypes were not predictive of any measures in experimentally inoculated adults.[50,52] Furthermore, in contrast to experimentally-inoculated adults, TNF-α genotype was not predictive of any outcomes measured in children.[50] Any discrepancy in outcomes of these 2 studies regarding the predictability of specific cytokine genotypes may be related to several factors, including patient age, natural versus experimental infection, polymorphisms being examined, severity of illness in individual subjects, and differences in the outcome measures themselves. Furthermore, cytokine responses are influenced by genotype and cellular signaling at transcriptional, translational, and post-translational levels, all potentially altering cytokine levels.

Other Mediators

It has also been suggested that viruses can trigger illness using local inflammatory mediators in addition to the cytokines produced during the systemic immune response. RSV infection and resulting antigen-antibody complexes stimulate a significant thromboxane B2 response from neutrophils, which may contribute to bronchoconstriction and superoxide, potentially implicating oxidative damage as a mediator of pathogenesis,[53] all of which may be COX-2 mediated.[54] Healthy adults experimentally inoculated with RSV who develop infection have a significant increase in leukotriene (LT) C_4, and there is an observed temporal relationship between the rising levels and the development of illness.[54] LTC_4 has been implicated as an important mediator in asthma pathogenesis.[55,56] However, although arachidonic acid pathway products have been shown to be upregulated with RSV infection,[54] in vitro, prostaglandin E_2 levels were not increased with RSV-infection of human alveolar mononuclear phagocytes.[57] Although nitric oxide (NO) has been recognized as an inflammatory mediator in lower and upper respiratory tract infections[58] and in vitro infection of epithelial cells produced increased nitrites and inducible NO synthase (iNOS),[59] healthy adults inoculated with RSV who later developed symptoms and had evidence of RSV infection did not have changes in NO levels,[60] which parallels studies done previously with influenza and rhinovirus.[61,62]

In Vitro Epithelial Cell Responses to RSV

The epithelium of the airway has been demonstrated to be important in immune signaling in RSV infection, by releasing chemokines responsible for initial signaling to inflammatory cells. RSV-infected bronchial epithelial cells show enhanced ICAM-1 expression that is thought to be autocrine in nature and mediated by IL-1α.[63] IL-8 has been demonstrated to be constitutively expressed by nasal epithelium but also upregulated with RSV infection.[64] RSV infection induces activator protein-1 (AP-1), nuclear factor IL-6 (NF-IL6), and NF-κB transcription and translation, which lead to upregulation of IL-8 production by epithelial cells.[65–67] Early studies of infection of bronchial epithelial cells with RSV showed that IL-8 production was detectable within 4 hours and accumulating in supernatants at 24 hours, whereas IL-6 and granulocyte macrophage colony-stimulating factor were present 96 hours after RSV infection, the phase of replication for the virus.[68] RSV infection of well-differentiated respiratory epithelial cells results in significant release of IL-8 and RANTES by 48 hours to the basolateral surface and probably influences the recruitment of leukocytes to sites of infection.[69] These chemokines can be substantially, but not completely, inhibited by administering inhaled corticosteroids,[70] possibly explaining the mechanism by which inhaled steroids benefit asthmatics during virus-induced exacerbations. A similar study demonstrated significant increase of RANTES after RSV-inoculation in an infection-dependent manner, and a similar effect was seen in vivo when comparing infected children with controls and asymptomatic baseline.[71]

IMMUNE RESPONSE TO RSV INFECTION IN ADULTS WITH ASTHMA

In examining the immunologic responses of asthmatics to RSV, there were differences when compared with healthy adult responses, as described in the previous section. In one study, adults asthmatics had reduced levels of IFN-α production by blood cells compared with matched controls when stimulated with RSV,[72] which represents an altered systemic response and not just a local cytokine response. Adults with acute asthma exacerbations and viral infection, including RSV, had increased levels of IL-10 compared with nonasthmatics with viral infections and stable asthmatics without infection.[73] However, although RANTES and MIP-1α mRNA were elevated with viral infection as mentioned earlier, this response was seen in asthmatics and nonasthmatics, suggesting that it may be more a reflection of the viral infection and not a response specific to asthmatics.[73] One interpretation of this data is that increased IL-10 gene expression may be responsible for suppressed eosinophil translocation in acute asthma exacerbations, because IL-10 has previously been shown to have an antieosinophilic effect in mouse models.[74] In children and adolescents with asthma, asthma severity has been correlated with IgG_1 and IgG_2 to G protein of RSV,[75] suggesting that these antibodies may play a direct role in airway hyperresponsiveness by activating complement or causing the release of histamine by cross-linking FcγRI receptors on mast cells.

In severe asthma exacerbations that resulted in death in which viral infection was established by PCR (3 rhinovirus, 2 RSV), higher percentages of activated (CD25+) CD8+ cells were present in postmortem lung samples than in nonasthmatics or asthmatics whose cause of death was unrelated to asthma.[76] Additionally, perforin expression, a marker of cytotoxicity, was highest in the fatal asthmatic group, and there was lower expression of bcl-2, an antiapoptotic gene, in both groups of asthmatics compared with controls. This may be evidence that the immune system permits apoptosis of virus-infected cells more readily in asthmatics, which may be a viral survival mechanism.[76] Furthermore, CD8+ production of IL-4 and IFN-γ was higher in the fatal asthmatic group than controls, with the IFN-γ/IL-4 ratio half the value found in controls,[76] which may support a T-cell switch phenomenon reported in viral infections that results in eosinophilia and impaired viral clearance.[77]

Another study demonstrated that the blood eosinophil count was higher in subjects with serologic evidence of current or recent RSV infection, further supporting the possible Th1/Th2 switch with RSV infection. Clinically, these subjects were more likely to be diagnosed with asthma by a physician or have bronchial hyperresponsiveness on provocative challenge.[78] In subjects with COPD undergoing serial RSV detection sampling, those who are more frequently infected have more rapid decline of lung function, independent of smoking status, frequency of exacerbation, or bacterial load in lower airways. The subjects with COPD also had more airway inflammation, measured by sputum IL-6, IL-8, and myeloperoxidase levels than those less frequently infected.[79] These markers of inflammation were associated with a trend to functional decline in FEV_1, potentially implicating a mechanism by which the virus may cause a decrease in FEV_1, but the investigators point out that the persistent inflammation could also predispose to RSV infection.

RESPONSE OF SPECIFIC CELL TYPES FROM ADULTS WITH ASTHMA TO RSV

Among the different cell types involved in the immune response, it has been postu-lated that RSV infections in asthmatics may elicit a different response from the same cells from RSV infections in nonasthmatics.[80] In vitro RSV infection of PBMCs revealed that although the cytokines IL-6 and IL-10 that are associated with innate immunity did not differ between asthmatics and nonasthmatics, the adaptive immune response of asthmatics showed a trend to stronger IFN-γ production and significantly decreased IL-13. Neutralizing IL-10 had no impact on the response, supporting the idea that the trend was not due to counter-regulation by IL-10.[80] Furthermore, block-ing toll-like receptor 4, which had been implicated in RSV-mediated cytokine release in mice,[81] did not abrogate RSV-stimulated IL-6 or IFN-γ.

IMMUNE RESPONSES TO OTHER ANTIGENS INFLUENCED BY RSV INFECTION

Conjecture and evidence support RSV infection also indirectly contributing to illness in asthmatics and asthma exacerbations by upregulating immune responses to other antigens. For instance, adults experimentally inoculated with RSV have increased wheal and flare responses and new positive allergen responses measurable as late as 21 days after exposure.[82] In seeming contrast to these in vivo findings, PBMCs from atopic adults had increased IL-5 production when exposed to mite allergen, but this was attenuated with live RSV infection for which these subjects showed signif-icantly higher IFN-γ production compared with nonatopic subjects.[83] Similarly, the PMBCs from atopic asthmatic subjects had a sixfold increase in the frequency of IL-4-producing cells to cat and birch allergen compared with nonasthmatics; however, atopic subjects had significantly more IFN-γ-producing cells specific for the RSV F/G proteins than nonatopics.[84] Additionally, inactivated RSV increased IL-10 production in atopic subjects' PBMCs when concurrently exposed to mite allergen, further demonstrating the influence of RSV exposure to immune responses of mite allergen in atopic subjects.[83]

DOES EARLY-LIFE RSV INFECTION CONTRIBUTE TO ASTHMA IN ADULTS?

One question that has persisted, regardless of any data supporting RSV's role in morbidity in adult asthmatics, is the existence of a causative role for RSV infection early in life in determining the presence of asthma in adulthood. One longitudinal case-control study of children hospitalized for RSV bronchiolitis in infancy revealed an increased prevalence of asthma up to age 13 years compared with controls hospitalized for other reasons.[1] Continued follow-up of this Swedish population will be very informative about the long-term risk of severe infant RSV bronchiolitis for adult asthma. In a study in Arizona of children who experienced lower respiratory tract viral infection, yet who were not hospitalized, RSV infection in early life was significantly associated with wheezing up to age 11 years but not beyond.[2] Very few studies to date have followed subjects long enough to be informative about RSV infection in childhood and the subsequent risk of developing asthma. In a long-term follow-up of infants hospitalized with bronchiolitis, a multivariate analysis demonstrated that elevated eosinophils outside of infection predicted recurrent wheezing only until early school years but not into adulthood.[85] Subjects infected with RSV had lower eosinophil counts during infection than those with non-RSV bronchiolitis, but during convalescence, there was no difference in eosinophil counts.[85] In a subgroup analysis of these same subjects, a non-RSV cause of bronchiolitis was a significant risk factor of asthma in adulthood compared with those with RSV-associated bronchiolitis as infants, with no significant difference between the 2 groups when examining lung function, although the power of study was fairly low.[86] A separate analysis of this same cohort showed that although RSV bronchiolitis was an independent risk factor of lung-function testing abnormality, it was not associated with asthma or bronchial reactivity in adulthood when controlling for atopy diagnosed by at least one positive skin prick test, and atopy was similar between the RSV-infected and controls.[87] These results suggest that RSV bronchiolitis in infancy does not directly predispose one to asthma and/or atopy; instead, it may represent a marker of common abnormalities seen in both conditions related to immune function.[88] However, the investigators do correctly point out that the power of their study is limited by more subjects in the cohort dropping out than meeting the diagnostic criteria used for asthma. Therefore, continued follow-up of the cohorts from Sweden and Arizona must be done to more fully determine the relationship between RSV infection in infancy and the development of asthma.

IMMUNE SUBVERSION BY RSV

RSV has various different mechanisms by which it can suppress the host antiviral immune response and therefore aid its own survival. Two major RSV proteins that antagonize host defense are the nonstructural (NS) proteins, NS1 and NS2.[89] There are 2 promoter proximal genes that code for these 2 proteins, which are termed nonstructural because they are synthesized in RSV-infected cells but not packaged in the mature virion structure.[89] The predicted structures of NS1 and NS2 do not share any significant homology with any other protein.[89] Recombinant RSV strains have been created in which either or both NS genes have been deleted to determine how these NS proteins regulate immune evasion. To fully understand the methods by which the 2 RSV NS proteins subvert host immunity, a brief review of antiviral host defense is necessary.

RSV binds to the cell membrane through its G protein, which is the attachment protein.[89] The RSV F protein is the fusion protein that allows for the virus to penetrate the cell membrane.[89] Once in the cell, RNA viruses, such as RSV, can be recognized by RNA helicases that include retinoic acid inducible gene I (RIG-I), melanoma differentiation associated gene 5 (MDA5), and laboratory of genetics and physiology 2 (LGP2).[90] RNA recognition by RIG-I requires the presence of a free 5'-triphosphate structure and this allows for differentiation of nonself viral RNA from self RNA, because host RNA is either capped or post-translationally modified to remove the 5'-triphosphate.[91] Because of this requirement for the 5'-triphosphate structure for RIG-I recognition, viruses that activate RIG-I include RSV and related paramyxoviruses, such as human metapneumovirus, as well as influenza A.[91] RIG-I and MDA5 contain 2 N-terminal caspase activation and recruitment domains (CARDs) that are essential for their signaling activity.[90] After binding the nonself ligand, RIG-I and MDA5 interact via these CARD domains with the signaling-adaptor molecule IFN-β promoter stimulator 1 (IPS-1) that is present in the outer mitochondrial membrane.[90] Experiments using an NS2-deletion RSV revealed NS2-inhibited RIG-I-mediated IFN promoter activation by binding to the N-terminal CARD of RIG-I, thus blocking its interaction with the downstream component IPS-1.[92] IPS-1 recruits a signaling complex to activate transcription factors, including interferon regulatory factor (IRF3) and NF-κB. Activated IRF-3 and NF-κB can translocate to the nucleus, resulting in induced expression of the Type I IFNs, IFN-α and IFN-β, as well as IRF3 target genes and NF-κB target genes to drive antiviral and inflammatory responses against infection.[90]

Other experiments revealed that NS2 is essential for the early inhibition of IFN transcription, because infection with the NS2-deletion mutant of RSV resulted in a greater level of IRF3 compared with wild-type RSV containing NS2.[92] Experiments using an RSV deficient in NS1 indicated that this protein also negatively regulated IRF3 activation by reducing IKKε, an important protein kinase that phosphorylates and activates IRF3.[93] Thus, RSV NS1 prevented IRF-3 translocation to the nucleus by inhibiting IRF-3 phosphorylation and activation, blocking Type I IFN production. Other experiments revealed that NS1 and NS2 acted cooperatively to suppress IRF-3 activation and, therefore, its nuclear translocation.[94] Type I IFN production can also be blocked further downstream as the NS1/NS2 heterodimeric complex upregulates expression of suppressor of cytokine signaling (SOCS) 1, which also inhibited Type I IFN production.[95]

After the Type I IFNs are produced by the cell, they can act in an autocrine or paracrine fashion to stimulate cellular antiviral defense by binding to the same heterodimeric IFN-α/-β receptor, resulting in activation of Tyk2 and Jak1 and phosphorylation of the cytoplasmic transcription factors, signal transducer and activator of transcription (STAT)1 and STAT2.[91] IRF9 is recruited to the phosphorylated STAT1/STAT2 heterodimer to form the IFN-stimulated gene factor 3 (ISGF3) heterotrimeric complex, which can translocate to the nucleus and induce transcription of the Type I IFN-regulated genes.[91] RSV can interrupt this pathway at several different points. For instance, both NS1 and NS2 degrade STAT2 to inhibit Type I IFN signaling.[93,96,97] The NS1 protein used the elongin-cullin E3 ligase to target proteasomal degradation of STAT2.[98]

The NS proteins affect production of antiviral IFN proteins and subvert host defense by other mechanisms as well. Experiments using RSV in which NS1 was deleted resulted in augmented expression of dendritic cell surface markers that are characteristic of maturation, in addition to heightened expression of several chemokines and cytokines. Although deletion of NS2 by itself did not have an effect on these endpoints, deletion of NS2 and NS1 further increased the effects present with NS1 deletion alone.[99] These results suggest that NS1 decreases dendritic cell maturation and cytokine secretion and is aided in this activity by NS2. NS proteins also inhibited cell apoptosis of infected cells by expressing several antiapoptotic factors, allowing for greater viral replication and subsequent release of viral progeny. Experiments using short interfering RNAs (siRNA) for NS1 and NS2 led to a reduction in the expression of antiapoptotic proteins, resulting in early cell death and a significant decrease in RSV growth.[100] Finally, NS2 suppresses cytotoxic T lymphocyte responses. Mouse experiments using an RSV in which NS2 was deleted resulted in a greater RSV-specific cytotoxic T lymphocyte response in the lung, an increase in IFN-γ-producing CD8 cells, and cytotoxicity.[101]

SUMMARY

Through epidemiologic studies, RSV is increasingly recognized as an important cause of asthma exacerbations in adults, especially in the elderly. The phenotypic response to RSV infection at the molecular, the cellular, and the individual subject level can be explained at least partly by the immunologic milieu of the host at the time of infection, which depends on host gene-environment interactions and is manifested in the different cytokine and cellular responses between asthmatics and nonasthmatics. Whether severe early-life RSV infection contributes to asthma persisting into adulthood is unknown, but ongoing longitudinal studies may provide clues as to whether this is the case. Finally, RSV has unique capabilities for subverting host antiviral responses, and understanding these mechanisms may provide novel therapeutic targets against this important pathogen.

REFERENCES

1. Sigurs N, Gustafsson PM, Bjarnason R, et al. Severe respiratory syncytial virus bronchiolitis in infancy and asthma and allergy at age 13. Am J Respir Crit Care Med 2005;171(2):137–41.
2. Stein RT, Sherrill D, Morgan WJ, et al. Respiratory syncytial virus in early life and risk of wheeze and allergy by age 13 years. Lancet 1999;354(9178):541–5 [see comments].
3. Falsey AR, Hennessey PA, Formica MA, et al. Respiratory syncytial virus infection in elderly and high-risk adults. N Engl J Med 2005;352(17):1749–59.
4. Beasley R, Coleman ED, Hermon Y, et al. Viral respiratory tract infection and exacerbations of asthma in adult patients. Thorax 1988;43(9):679–83.
5. Glezen WP, Greenberg SB, Atmar RL, et al. Impact of respiratory virus infections on persons with chronic underlying conditions. JAMA 2000;283(4):499–505.
6. Harju TH, Leinonen M, Nokso-Koivisto J, et al. Pathogenic bacteria and viruses in induced sputum or pharyngeal secretions of adults with stable asthma. Thorax 2006;61(7):579–84.
7. Teichtahl H, Buckmaster N, Pertnikovs E. The incidence of respiratory tract infection in adults requiring hospitalization for asthma. Chest 1997;112(3): 591–6.
8. Nicholson KG, Kent J, Ireland DC. Respiratory viruses and exacerbations of asthma in adults. BMJ 1993;307(6910):982–6.
9. Sokhandan M, McFadden ERJ, Huang YT, et al. The contribution of respiratory viruses to severe exacerbations of asthma in adults. Chest 1995;107(6):1570–4 [see comments].
10. Ayres JG, Noah ND, Fleming DM. Incidence of episodes of acute asthma and acute bronchitis in general practice 1976–87. Br J Gen Pract 1993;43(374): 361–4.
11. Pattemore PK, Johnston SL, Bardin PG. Viruses as precipitants of asthma symptoms. I. Epidemiology. Clin Exp Allergy 1992;22(3):325–36.
12. Abramson M, Pearson L, Kutin J, et al. Allergies, upper respiratory tract infections, and asthma. J Asthma 1994;31(5):367–74.
13. Dowell SF, Anderson LJ, Gary HEJ, et al. Respiratory syncytial virus is an important cause of community- acquired lower respiratory infection among hospitalized adults. J Infect Dis 1996;174(3):456–62.
14. Fleming DM, Cross KW. Respiratory syncytial virus or influenza? Lancet 1993; 342(8886–8887):1507–10.

15. Griffin MR, Coffey CS, Neuzil KM, et al. Winter viruses: influenza- and respiratory syncytial virus-related morbidity in chronic lung disease. Arch Intern Med 2002; 162(11):1229–36.
16. Hall CB, Long CE, Schnabel KC. Respiratory syncytial virus infections in previously healthy working adults. Clin Infect Dis 2001;33(6):792–6.
17. Moineddin R, Nie JX, Domb G, et al. Seasonality of primary care utilization for respiratory diseases in Ontario: a time-series analysis. BMC Health Serv Res 2008;8:160.
18. Thompson WW, Shay DK, Weintraub E, et al. Mortality associated with influenza and respiratory syncytial virus in the United States. JAMA 2003;289(2):179–86.
19. Zambon MC, Stockton JD, Clewley JP, et al. Contribution of influenza and respiratory syncytial virus to community cases of influenza-like illness: an observational study. Lancet 2001;358(9291):1410–6.
20. Guidry GG, Black-Payne CA, Payne DK, et al. Respiratory syncytial virus infection among intubated adults in a university medical intensive care unit. Chest 1991;100(5):1377–84.
21. Duncan CB, Walsh EE, Peterson DR, et al. Risk factors for respiratory failure associated with respiratory syncytial virus infection in adults. J Infect Dis 2009;200(8):1242–6.
22. Gill MA, Palucka AK, Barton T, et al. Mobilization of plasmacytoid and myeloid dendritic cells to mucosal sites in children with respiratory syncytial virus and other viral respiratory infections. J Infect Dis 2005;191(7):1105–15.
23. Gill MA, Long K, Kwon T, et al. Differential recruitment of dendritic cells and monocytes to respiratory mucosal sites in children with influenza virus or respiratory syncytial virus infection. J Infect Dis 2008;198(11):1667–76.
24. Henderson FW, Collier AM, Clyde WA Jr, et al. Respiratory-syncytial-virus infections, reinfections and immunity. A prospective, longitudinal study in young children. N Engl J Med 1979;300(10):530–4.
25. Popow-Kraupp T, Lakits E, Kellner G, et al. Immunoglobulin-class-specific immune response to respiratory syncytial virus structural proteins in infants, children, and adults. J Med Virol 1989;27(3):215–23.
26. Falsey AR, Singh HK, Walsh EE. Serum antibody decay in adults following natural respiratory syncytial virus infection. J Med Virol 2006;78(11):1493–7.
27. Lee FE, Walsh EE, Falsey AR, et al. Experimental infection of humans with A2 respiratory syncytial virus. Antiviral Res 2004;63(3):191–6.
28. Mills J, Van Kirk JE, Wright PF, et al. Experimental respiratory syncytial virus infection of adults. Possible mechanisms of resistance to infection and illness. J Immunol 1971;107(1):123–30.
29. Walsh EE, Falsey AR. Humoral and mucosal immunity in protection from natural respiratory syncytial virus infection in adults. J Infect Dis 2004;190(2):373–8.
30. Hall CB, Walsh EE, Long CE, et al. Immunity to and frequency of reinfection with respiratory syncytial virus. J Infect Dis 1991;163(4):693–8.
31. Falsey AR, Walsh EE, Looney RJ, et al. Comparison of respiratory syncytial virus humoral immunity and response to infection in young and elderly adults. J Med Virol 1999;59(2):221–6.
32. Walsh EE, Falsey AR. Age related differences in humoral immune response to respiratory syncytial virus infection in adults. J Med Virol 2004;73(2):295–9.
33. Falsey AR, McCann RM, Hall WJ, et al. Acute respiratory tract infection in daycare centers for older persons. J Am Geriatr Soc 1995;43(1):30–6.
34. Gardner EM, Murasko DM. Age-related changes in Type 1 and Type 2 cytokine production in humans. Biogerontology 2002;3(5):271–90.

35. Looney RJ, Falsey AR, Walsh E, et al. Effect of aging on cytokine production in response to respiratory syncytial virus infection. J Infect Dis 2002;185(5):682–5.

36. Po JL, Gardner EM, Anaraki F, et al. Age-associated decrease in virus-specific CD8+ T lymphocytes during primary influenza infection. Mech Ageing Dev 2002;123(8):1167–81.

37. Zhang Y, Luxon BA, Casola A, et al. Expression of respiratory syncytial virus-induced chemokine gene networks in lower airway epithelial cells revealed by cDNA microarrays. J Virol 2001;75(19):9044–58.

38. Falsey AR, Walsh EE. Humoral immunity to respiratory syncytial virus infection in the elderly. J Med Virol 1992;36(1):39–43.

39. Walsh EE, Peterson DR, Falsey AR. Risk factors for severe respiratory syncytial virus infection in elderly persons. J Infect Dis 2004;189(2):233–8.

40. Terrosi C, Di GG, Martorelli B, et al. Humoral immunity to respiratory syncytial virus in young and elderly adults. Epidemiol Infect 2009;137(12):1684–6.

41. Ostler T, Davidson W, Ehl S. Virus clearance and immunopathology by CD8(+) T cells during infection with respiratory syncytial virus are mediated by IFN-gamma. Eur J Immunol 2002;32(8):2117–23.

42. Cherrie AH, Anderson K, Wertz GW, et al. Human cytotoxic T cells stimulated by antigen on dendritic cells recognize the N, SH, F, M, 22K, and 1b proteins of respiratory syncytial virus. J Virol 1992;66(4):2102–10.

43. Lee FE, Walsh EE, Falsey AR, et al. The balance between influenza- and RSV-specific CD4 T cells secreting IL-10 or IFNgamma in young and healthy-elderly subjects. Mech Ageing Dev 2005;126(11):1223–9.

44. Effros RB. Replicative senescence of CD8 T cells: effect on human ageing. Exp Gerontol 2004;39(4):517–24.

45. de Bree GJ, Heidema J, van Leeuwen EM, et al. Respiratory syncytial virus-specific CD8+ memory T cell responses in elderly persons. J Infect Dis 2005; 191(10):1710–8.

46. Anderson LJ, Tsou C, Potter C, et al. Cytokine response to respiratory syncytial virus stimulation of human peripheral blood mononuclear cells. J Infect Dis 1994;170(5):1201–8.

47. Noah TL, Becker S. Chemokines in nasal secretions of normal adults experimentally infected with respiratory syncytial virus. Clin Immunol 2000;97(1):43–9.

48. Groskreutz DJ, Monick MM, Powers LS, et al. Respiratory syncytial virus induces TLR3 protein and protein kinase R, leading to increased double-stranded RNA responsiveness in airway epithelial cells. J Immunol 2006;176(3):1733–40.

49. Zhang Y, Wang Y, Gilmore X, et al. An aged mouse model for RSV infection and diminished CD8(+) CTL responses. Exp Biol Med (Maywood) 2002;227(2): 133–40.

50. Gentile DA, Doyle WJ, Zeevi A, et al. Cytokine gene polymorphisms moderate illness severity in infants with respiratory syncytial virus infection. Hum Immunol 2003;64(3):338–44.

51. Gentile DA, Doyle WJ, Zeevi A, et al. Cytokine gene polymorphisms moderate responses to respiratory syncytial virus in adults. Hum Immunol 2003;64(1): 93–8.

52. Genovese M, Van den Bosch F, Roberson S, et al. LY2439821, a humanized anti-IL-17 monoclonal antibody, in the treatment of patients with rheumatoid arthritis. Arthritis Rheum 2010;62(4):929–39.

53. Faden H, Kaul TN, Ogra PL. Activation of oxidative and arachidonic acid metabolism in neutrophils by respiratory syncytial virus antibody complexes: possible role in disease. J Infect Dis 1983;148(1):110–6.

54. Richardson JY, Ottolini MG, Pletneva L, et al. Respiratory syncytial virus (RSV) infection induces cyclooxygenase 2: a potential target for RSV therapy. J Immunol 2005;174(7):4356–64.

55. Henderson WR Jr, Lewis DB, Albert RK, et al. The importance of leukotrienes in airway inflammation in a mouse model of asthma. J Exp Med 1996;184(4): 1483–94.

56. Henderson WR Jr, Tang LO, Chu SJ, et al. A role for cysteinyl leukotrienes in airway remodeling in a mouse asthma model. Am J Respir Crit Care Med 2002;165(1):108–16.

57. Panuska JR, Midulla F, Cirino NM, et al. Virus-induced alterations in macrophage production of tumor necrosis factor and prostaglandin E2. Am J Physiol 1990; 259(6 Pt 1):L396–402.

58. Hart CM. Nitric oxide in adult lung disease. Chest 1999;115(5):1407–17.

59. Kao YJ, Piedra PA, Larsen GL, et al. Induction and regulation of nitric oxide synthase in airway epithelial cells by respiratory syncytial virus. Am J Respir Crit Care Med 2001;163(2):532–9.

60. Gentile DA, Doyle WJ, Belenky S, et al. Nasal and oral nitric oxide levels during experimental respiratory syncytial virus infection of adults. Acta Otolaryngol 2002;122(1):61–6.

61. Kaul P, Singh I, Turner RB. Effect of nitric oxide on rhinovirus replication and virus-induced interleukin-8 elaboration. Am J Respir Crit Care Med 1999; 159(4 Pt 1):1193–8.

62. Murphy AW, Platts-Mills TA, Lobo M, et al. Respiratory nitric oxide levels in experimental human influenza. Chest 1998;114(2):452–6.

63. Patel JA, Kunimoto M, Sim TC, et al. Interleukin-1 alpha mediates the enhanced expression of intercellular adhesion molecule-1 in pulmonary epithelial cells infected with respiratory syncytial virus. Am J Respir Cell Mol Biol 1995;13(5): 602–9.

64. Becker S, Koren HS, Henke DC. Interleukin-8 expression in normal nasal epithelium and its modulation by infection with respiratory syncytial virus and cytokines tumor necrosis factor, interleukin-1, and interleukin-6. Am J Respir Cell Mol Biol 1993;8(1):20–7.

65. Jamaluddin M, Garofalo R, Ogra PL, et al. Inducible translational regulation of the NF-IL6 transcription factor by respiratory syncytial virus infection in pulmonary epithelial cells. J Virol 1996;70(3):1554–63.

66. Mastronarde JG, He B, Monick MM, et al. Induction of interleukin (IL)-8 gene expression by respiratory syncytial virus involves activation of nuclear factor (NF)-kappa B and NF-IL-6. J Infect Dis 1996;174(2):262–7.

67. Mastronarde JG, Monick MM, Mukaida N, et al. Activator protein-1 is the preferred transcription factor for cooperative interaction with nuclear factor-kappaB in respiratory syncytial virus-induced interleukin-8 gene expression in airway epithelium. J Infect Dis 1998;177(5):1275–81.

68. Noah TL, Becker S. Respiratory syncytial virus-induced cytokine production by a human bronchial epithelial cell line. Am J Physiol 1993;265(5 Pt 1): L472–8.

69. Mellow TE, Murphy PC, Carson JL, et al. The effect of respiratory synctial virus on chemokine release by differentiated airway epithelium. Exp Lung Res 2004; 30(1):43–57.

70. Noah TL, Wortman IA, Becker S. The effect of fluticasone propionate on respiratory syncytial virus-induced chemokine release by a human bronchial epithelial cell line. Immunopharmacology 1998;39(3):193–9.

71. Becker S, Reed W, Henderson FW, et al. RSV infection of human airway epithelial cells causes production of the beta-chemokine RANTES. Am J Physiol 1997; 272(3 Pt 1):L512–20.

72. Gehlhar K, Bilitewski C, Reinitz-Rademacher K, et al. Impaired virus-induced interferon-alpha2 release in adult asthmatic patients. Clin Exp Allergy 2006; 36(3):331–7.

73. Grissell TV, Powell H, Shafren DR, et al. Interleukin-10 gene expression in acute virus-induced asthma. Am J Respir Crit Care Med 2005;172(4):433–9.

74. van Scott MR, Justice JP, Bradfield JF, et al. IL-10 reduces Th2 cytokine production and eosinophilia but augments airway reactivity in allergic mice. Am J Physiol Lung Cell Mol Physiol 2000;278(4):L667–74.

75. Hancock GE, Scheuer CA, Sierzega R, et al. Adaptive immune responses of patients with asthma to the attachment (G) glycoprotein of respiratory synctial virus. J Infect Dis 2001;184(12):1589–93.

76. O'Sullivan S, Cormican L, Faul JL, et al. Activated, cytotoxic CD8(+) T lymphocytes contribute to the pathology of asthma death. Am J Respir Crit Care Med 2001;164(4):560–4.

77. Coyle AJ, Erard F, Bertrand C, et al. Virus-specific CD8+ cells can switch to interleukin 5 production and induce airway eosinophilia. J Exp Med 1995; 181(3):1229–33.

78. Bjornsson E, Hjelm E, Janson C, et al. Serology of respiratory viruses in relation to asthma and bronchial hyperresponsiveness. Ups J Med Sci 1996;101(2): 159–68.

79. Wilkinson TM, Donaldson GC, Johnston SL, et al. Respiratory syncytial virus, airway inflammation, and FEV1 decline in patients with chronic obstructive pulmonary disease. Am J Respir Crit Care Med 2006;173(8):871–6.

80. Douville RN, Bastien N, Li Y, et al. Adult asthmatics display exaggerated IFNgamma responses to human metapneumovirus and respiratory syncytial virus. Biochem Cell Biol 2007;85(2):252–8.

81. Haynes LM, Moore DD, Kurt-Jones EA, et al. Involvement of toll-like receptor 4 in innate immunity to respiratory syncytial virus. J Virol 2001;75(22):10730–7.

82. Skoner DP, Gentile DA, Angelini B, et al. Allergy skin test responses during experimental infection with respiratory syncytial virus. Ann Allergy Asthma Immunol 2006;96(6):834–9.

83. Hirose H, Matsuse H, Tsuchida T, et al. Cytokine production from peripheral blood mononuclear cells of mite allergen-sensitized atopic adults stimulated with respiratory syncytial virus and mite allergen. Int Arch Allergy Immunol 2008;146(2):149–55.

84. Pala P, Message SD, Johnston SL, et al. Increased aeroallergen-specific interleukin-4-producing T cells in asthmatic adults. Clin Exp Allergy 2002;32(12): 1739–44.

85. Piippo-Savolainen E, Remes S, Korppi M. Does blood eosinophilia in wheezing infants predict later asthma? A prospective 18-20-year follow-up. Allergy Asthma Proc 2007;28(2):163–9.

86. Piippo-Savolainen E, Korppi M, Korhonen K, et al. Adult asthma after non-respiratory syncytial virus bronchiolitis in infancy: subgroup analysis of the 20-year prospective follow-up study. Pediatr Int 2007;49(2):190–5.

87. Korppi M, Piippo-Savolainen E, Korhonen K, et al. Respiratory morbidity 20 years after RSV infection in infancy. Pediatr Pulmonol 2004;38(2):155–60.

88. Welliver RC. Immunologic mechanisms of virus-induced wheezing and asthma [review]. J Pediatr 1999;135(2 Pt 2):14–20.

89. Collins PL, Crowe JE Jr. Respiratory syncytial virus and metapneumovirus. In: Knipe DM, Howley PM, editors. Fields virology. 5th edition. Philadelphia: Lippincott Williams & Wilkins; 2007. p. 1602–41.
90. Takeuchi O, Akira S. MDA5/RIG-I and virus recognition. Curr Opin Immunol 2008;20(1):17–22.
91. Wilkins C, Gale M Jr. Recognition of viruses by cytoplasmic sensors. Curr Opin Immunol 2010;22(1):41–7.
92. Ling Z, Tran KC, Teng MN. Human respiratory syncytial virus nonstructural protein NS2 antagonizes the activation of beta interferon transcription by interacting with RIG-I. J Virol 2009;83(8):3734–42.
93. Swedan S, Musiyenko A, Barik S. Respiratory syncytial virus nonstructural proteins decrease levels of multiple members of the cellular interferon pathways. J Virol 2009;83(19):9682–93.
94. Spann KM, Tran KC, Collins PL. Effects of nonstructural proteins NS1 and NS2 of human respiratory syncytial virus on interferon regulatory factor 3, NF-kappaB, and proinflammatory cytokines. J Virol 2005;79(9):5353–62.
95. Moore EC, Barber J, Tripp RA. Respiratory syncytial virus (RSV) attachment and nonstructural proteins modify the type I interferon response associated with suppressor of cytokine signaling (SOCS) proteins and IFN-stimulated gene-15 (ISG15). Virol J 2008;5:116.
96. Lo MS, Brazas RM, Holtzman MJ. Respiratory syncytial virus nonstructural proteins NS1 and NS2 mediate inhibition of Stat2 expression and alpha/beta interferon responsiveness. J Virol 2005;79(14):9315–9.
97. Ramaswamy M, Shi L, Varga SM, et al. Respiratory syncytial virus nonstructural protein 2 specifically inhibits type I interferon signal transduction. Virology 2006; 344(2):328–39.
98. Elliott J, Lynch OT, Suessmuth Y, et al. Respiratory syncytial virus NS1 protein degrades STAT2 by using the Elongin-Cullin E3 ligase. J Virol 2007;81(7): 3428–36.
99. Munir S, Le NC, Luongo C, et al. Nonstructural proteins 1 and 2 of respiratory syncytial virus suppress maturation of human dendritic cells. J Virol 2008; 82(17):8780–96.
100. Bitko V, Shulyayeva O, Mazumder B, et al. Nonstructural proteins of respiratory syncytial virus suppress premature apoptosis by an NF-kappaB-dependent, interferon-independent mechanism and facilitate virus growth. J Virol 2007; 81(4):1786–95.
101. Kotelkin A, Bolyakov IM, Yang L, et al. The NS2 protein of human respiratory syncytial virus suppresses the cytotoxic T-cell response as a consequence of suppressing the type I interferon response. J Virol 2006;80(12):5958–67.

New Human Rhinovirus Species and Their Significance in Asthma Exacerbation and Airway Remodeling

E. Kathryn Miller, MD, MPH

KEYWORDS

• Asthma • Rhinovirus • Bronchiolitis • Exacerbation

Asthma is the most common chronic disease of childhood, affecting 10% to 15% of all children.[1] Several different stimuli including allergens, tobacco smoke, certain drugs, and viral or bacterial infections are known to exacerbate asthma symptoms. Among these triggers, viruses are frequent inducers of asthma exacerbations, with human rhinoviruses (HRVs) being the most common in children and adults.[2–11] Moreover, HRVs are associated with a significant burden of lower respiratory tract disease,[2,12–15] and this may contribute to the development of asthma during infancy.[11,16]

HRV HISTORY

HRVs, which were first identified in culture in 1956, are members of the Picornaviridae family (pico, small; rna, RNA genome).[17,18] More than 100 serotypes of HRV have been identified to date.[17,19–21] HRVs are the most common cause of common cold in both adults and children. Although once thought to cause only common cold, it is now known that rhinoviruses are associated with lower respiratory tract illness.[4–6,11–15,22,23] In addition, HRV is an important cause of bronchiolitis, pneumonia, and otitis in infants and school-aged children.[24–26] During recent years, in studies using the more sensitive reverse transcriptase polymerase chain reaction (RT-PCR), HRVs have been associated with a significant burden of disease in infants and young children.[14,27] In one US population-based surveillance study of children younger than 5 years hospitalized with respiratory symptoms or fever, rhinovirus was detected

Conflict of interest: None.
Funding: KL2 RR24977-03, NIH; Thrasher.
Pediatric Pulmonary, Allergy and Immunology, Department of Pediatrics, Vanderbilt University Medical Center, Vanderbilt Children's Hospital, 11215 Doctors' Office Tower, 2200 Children's Way, Nashville, TN 37232-9500, USA
E-mail address: eva.k.miller@vanderbilt.edu

Immunol Allergy Clin N Am 30 (2010) 541–552
doi:10.1016/j.iac.2010.08.007
0889-8561/10/$ – see front matter © 2010 Elsevier Inc. All rights reserved.

in nasal/throat swabs by RT-PCR in 26%, representing 5 hospitalizations per 1000 children. HRV-associated hospitalization was more frequent in children younger than 6 months than in those aged 6 to 23 months or 24 to 59 months (17.6, 6.0, and 2.0 hospitalizations per 1000 children, respectively).[14] Rhinoviruses are best identified by RT-PCR performed on nasal secretions from infected individuals. However, not all rhinovirus infections are associated with symptoms. HRVs have been detected by RT-PCR in an average of 15% of asymptomatic individuals.[28]

HRVs are distributed worldwide with no predictable pattern of infection based on serotype. Multiple types may be present in a community or person at one time; HRV strains belonging to the same genetic cluster may be isolated during consecutive epidemic seasons, suggesting persistence in a community over an extended period. In temperate climates, the incidence of HRV infection peaks in fall, with another peak in spring, but HRV infections occur year-round.[29] Rhinoviruses are the major infectious trigger for asthma among young children, and studies have described a sharp increase in asthma exacerbations in this age group when school opens each fall (often referred to as the "September asthma epidemic").[30] Peak HRV incidence in the tropics occurs during the rainy season from June to October.

HRV AND ASTHMA

HRVs are the most common trigger of asthma exacerbations in children and adults.[2–11] In the study of population-based rates of HRV infection in children younger than 5 years hospitalized with respiratory symptoms or fever, infections were more frequent in children with a history of wheezing or asthma than in those without such a history (25 vs 3 hospitalizations per 1000 children). More than 80% of pediatric asthma is diagnosed before 5 years of age.[31] Bronchiolitis, a lower respiratory tract infection in infants presenting with wheezing, rales, and respiratory distress, has typically been associated with respiratory syncytial virus (RSV) infection,[15,16] but recent studies have identified HRVs as another important cause of bronchiolitis.[15,17–19] A study from Greece found that the presence of rhinovirus in bronchiolitis increased the risk for developing severe disease by almost 5-fold.[24] Bronchiolitis caused by RSV has been linked to the subsequent development of asthma.[12–14] HRV-related wheezing in infancy has also been hypothesized to play a causal role in the development of childhood asthma.[11,16] One study demonstrated that infants from atopic families with wheezing and HRV infection in the first 3 years of life have an increased likelihood of developing subsequent childhood asthma at the age of 6 years (odds ratio, 25.6). In this study, 90% of children who had wheezing and HRV when they were 3 years old had asthma at the age of 6 years.[11] Another study implicated HRV as a causative agent for asthma based on bronchiolitis occurring during the HRV season and subsequent diagnosis of childhood asthma, but did not include viral testing.[32] The association of HRV with bronchiolitis[7,12,14] and asthma exacerbations suggests that HRV may be associated with the inception of asthma.

Ongoing studies are investigating the role of the host response in HRV-related illness and comparing it to the effects of viral pathogenicity on asthma exacerbations. Both allergen exposure and elevated IgE levels predispose patients with asthma to more severe respiratory symptoms in response to HRV infection. Studies suggest that abnormalities in the host cellular response to viral infection that result in impaired apoptosis and increased viral replication may be responsible for the severe and prolonged symptoms typical of asthmatic individuals. These mechanisms have yet to be elucidated.

HRVC: A New Rhinovirus Species

In the past, some HRV strains were difficult to detect by conventional methods because they do not grow well in culture. In fact, recent studies suggest that there are many rhinoviruses that are not cultivatable but have significant correlation with clinical illness. Traditional methods of virus typing using immune antisera have identified about 100 serotypes, classified into HRVA and HRVB species based on genetic sequence similarity.[17,19–21] More recent PCR-based studies have discovered a novel group, HRVC (also called HRVA2, HRVNY, HRVQPM, and HRVX).[2,33–40] HRVC has been proposed as a new HRV species in the genus *Enterovirus* by the International Committee on Taxonomy of Viruses (http://talk.ictvonline.org/media/p/1035.aspx). HRVC contains a distinct subgroup of strains. Since the discovery of this new species of HRV, other related viruses have been identified from different countries of Africa, Asia, Australia, Europe, and North America.[2,33–40] In 2009, Palmenberg and colleagues[41] published complete genome sequences of all 99 previously known HRV serotypes and numerous novel strains, and sequence analysis demonstrates that the HRVC group comprises a genetically distinct species.[41] The analysis also identified a potential new group, HRVD (or a subgroup of HRVA). **Fig. 1** illustrates the genetic diversity of rhinoviruses detected in one study on hospitalized children. The novel group HRVC contributed to a substantial burden of HRV-related illness.

The identification of a novel group of HRVs and the finding that a significant proportion of HRV-related illness is attributable to these new HRVs raises the question of why these viruses were not identified previously. One reason seems to be the extreme difficulty in recovering viable virus. Thus far, several groups have been unable to recover these viruses in culture, despite numerous classical and nonclassical approaches.[2,15,17]

It is likely that HRVC has been circulating for some time and is not a newly emergent virus. An extensive search of HRV sequences published in GenBank before 2006 was unable to identify any sequence that belonged to the HRVC group (Miller and colleagues, unpublished data, 2009). One group reported the detection of a genetically similar virus in a specimen taken in New York in 2004[13] and another showed that these viruses have been circulating since at least 2002.[2] The author's group has detected HRVC in respiratory specimens that were collected 20 years ago (Miller and colleagues, unpublished data, 2010).

HRVC Frequency and Symptoms

During recent years, RT-PCR–based studies of HRV have shown that these viruses are associated with a substantial number of upper and lower respiratory tract illness in outpatients and hospitalized adults and children,[7,22–27,29–32] with evidence that HRVC accounts for a large proportion of this HRV-associated illness. HRVC has been detected in patients with symptoms including acute upper or lower respiratory tract illness, wheezing, bronchiolitis, asthma exacerbations, chronic obstructive pulmonary disease (COPD) exacerbations, pneumonia, lower respiratory tract infection, cold and flulike illness, fever, cough, rhinitis, nasal congestion, bronchitis, retractions, crackle, bronchopneumonia, dyspnea, otitis media, gastroesophageal reflux disease, pericarditis, poor appetite, and apparent life-threatening events.[42] In published studies on adults and children with respiratory symptoms who were tested for HRVC, the proportion of HRV attributable to HRVC ranged from 8% to 81%.[2,34,36,40,43–53] The overall frequency of HRV in published studies on adults and children with respiratory symptoms ranges from 2% to 20% (**Table 1**).[2,34,36,40,43–53] Like HRVA and HRVB, HRVC has also been detected in asymptomatic individuals.[51]

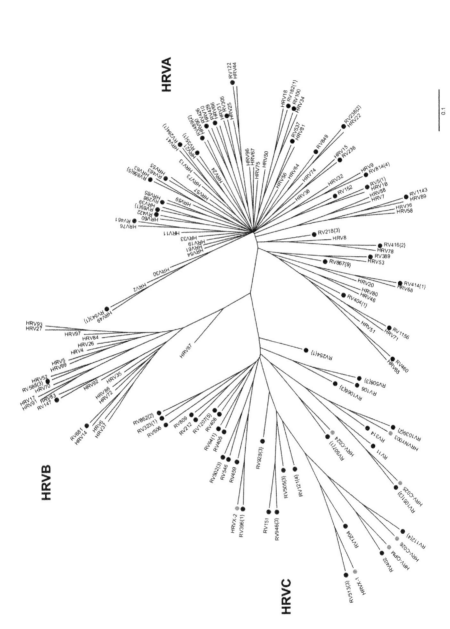

Fig. 1. Phylogenetic tree depicting relationships between known and novel HRV serotypes. Previously known HRV serotypes are designated by "HRV". Novel sequences identified in this study are designated by "RV" and a black circle. The numbers in braces after the label of these sequences indicate how many additional specimens contained each virus. Novel sequences identified in recent studies are designated by "HRV" and a gray circle.

Table 1
Summary of HRVC rates in studies of adults and children with acute respiratory tract illness based on inpatient versus outpatient status

	HRV+/Total Specimens (%)	HRVC/HRV Total (%)	Rates of HRVC (%)
Adults			
Inpatient	32	17	5
Outpatient	45	14	6
Children			
Inpatient	16–52	14–73	4–20
Outpatient	37	28	6
Mixed	13–22	8–81	2–10
Adults and Children, Inpatient and Outpatient	18	39	7
Overall	13–52	14–81	2–20[a]

[a] Overall prevalence of HRVC in published studies of adults and children with respiratory symptoms ranges from 2% to 20%.[2,29,31,36,38–41,43–48]

HRVC Seasonality

Among the studies that have tested for HRVC to date, data on seasonality of HRVC are not conclusive. Whereas many studies have detected HRVC as the predominant HRV species in the fall, suggesting that it may play a role in the so-called September asthma epidemic,[6,21,28] other studies in different regions and years have found otherwise. Han and colleagues[54] reported that HRVC was more common in the spring and HRVA in the fall in South Korea in 2006 but cocirculation occurred during both seasons. Consistent with the author's studies, Lau and colleagues[55] found HRVA and HRVC to alternate as the most common HRV species at different times during the peak seasons. Alternate disease activity by species and seasons suggests possible viral interference or serologic cross-protection between HRVA and HRVC.[55]

Whereas one study reported HRVC year-round without peaks in the spring and fall,[51] most studies do suggest that HRV species vary by season, year, and geographic location. This variation underscores the importance of studies over multiple years and seasons to understand fully the geographic and seasonal rhinovirus epidemiology.

Asymptomatic Infection with HRVC

It is clear that HRV infection occurs in ill individuals and experimental inoculation of patients with HRV induces respiratory symptoms; however, asymptomatic HRV infection has been documented. The rates of asymptomatic infection have been little studied. One study that included asymptomatic controls identified HRVC more often in sick than in well patients, with HRV detected in only 3 of 93 asymptomatic individuals.[51] There is some evidence that HRVC may interfere with infection by other viruses.[56]

HRVC and Asthma/Wheezing

Certain viruses may pose a greater risk for severe disease and asthma. There is much data to support a relationship of HRVC with wheezing/asthma (**Table 2**), but whether the symptoms produced by HRVC differ from those produced by HRVA or HRVB

Table 2
Summary of HRVC in patients with wheezing, bronchiolitis, or asthma

Study Type	Patient Age	Study Dates	Sample Size	Wheezing/Asthma Status	Different From HRVA/B (P<.05)	References
Inpatient, outpatient Retrospective	<80 y	Jan 2003–Dec 2003	1244	Wheezing, persistent cough	—	38,39
Inpatient	<14 y	Jan 2004–Dec 2008	1555	Asthma, recurrent wheezing, bronchiolitis	No	57
Inpatient Retrospective	<18 y	Nov 2004–Oct 2005	26	Wheezing	—	36
Inpatient, outpatient	<18 y	Dec 2004–Jul 2005	44	Wheezing	—	48
Prospective case-control	≥2 y	Mar 2003–Feb 2004	29	Asthma exacerbation, lower FEV	A and C in cases	50
Inpatient, outpatient	<2 y	Jan 2004–Dec 2004	447 (93 controls)	Wheezing	No	51
Inpatient Retrospective	<11 y	Feb 2006–Feb 2007	289	Bronchiolitis, wheezing, asthma	Trend	45,46
Inpatient Prospective	<5 y	Dec 2001–Sep 2003	1052	Asthma	Yes	2
Inpatient, PICU	<18 y	Feb 2007–Oct 2007	43	Wheezing	—	53
Inpatient Retrospective	<14 y	Jan 2006–Dec 2006	470	Asthma exacerbation, bronchiolitis	—	54
Inpatient Retrospective	<12 y	Oct 2005–Mar 2007	500	Asthma, bronchiolitis	—	58
Inpatient Prospective	<5 y	Jan 2007–Mar 2007	728	Wheezing, supplemental O_2	Yes	52
Inpatient	2 wk–5 y	2003–2006	97	Bronchiolitis	No	40
Inpatient	<18 y, adults	Apr 2004–Mar 2005	1200	Asthma, COPD, febrile wheezing	No	55
Outpatient	>18 y	Fall 2001–Dec 2004	83	Asthma	—	34

Other signs and symptoms associated with HRVC in some studies, which are not included in this table, include pneumonia, lower respiratory tract infection, cold and flu/like illness, fever, cough, rhinitis, nasal congestion, bronchitis, retractions, crackle, bronchopneumonia, upper respiratory tract illness, dyspnea, otitis, gastroesophageal reflux disease, pericarditis, poor appetite, and apparent life-threatening events.

Abbreviations: FEV, forced expiratory volume; PICU, pediatric intensive care unit.

strains is uncertain. In 2007, 4 retrospective studies showed a possible association of HRVC with wheezing or bronchiolitis.[34,36,39,40] In these studies, however, the sample size was insufficient to detect statistically significant clinical differences between HRVC and other species. In 2009 a large, prospective population-based study of young hospitalized children in 2 United States cities over 2 years found several clinically significant differences among patients infected with HRVC compared with those infected with HRVA, the other predominant HRV species. Of note, children with HRVC were twice as likely to have a discharge diagnosis of asthma than those with HRVA, and children with HRVA were more likely to present with fever.[2] In a similar study published in 2009 on a population of children younger than 5 years hospitalized with fever or acute respiratory tract illness in Amman, Jordan, HRVC was significantly more often associated with wheezing and supplemental oxygen use than HRVA.[52] An unpublished case-control study of 400 school-aged children with asthma in Argentina found slightly more HRVC in asthmatic children with upper respiratory tract infection and wheezing than in those with upper respiratory tract infection and no wheezing ($P =$ .036) (Miller and colleagues, unpublished data, 2010). One retrospective study investigated hospitalized children younger than 11 years and found a trend for HRVC to be detected more in patients with underlying asthma ($P = .09$).[45] HRVC was the most prevalent HRV species in this Thai study population, and was detected in 22% of 50 children aged 4 to 23 months with first wheezing episode. There were also 2 patients in this study who had been admitted with 5 different episodes of acute respiratory tract infection and subsequent recurrent wheezing associated with HRVA and HRVC.[46]

Other studies have reported HRVC in patients with wheezing, bronchiolitis, or asthma, but these studies either did not compare or did not find a significant difference between HRVC and HRVA or HRVB. McErlean and colleagues[39] detected HRVC (then called HRVQPM) in 17 of 1244 (1.4%) ill adult and pediatric patients. HRVC was the sole virus detected in 62% of the patients, and patients with HRVC infection alone were sicker than those with coinfections. In this study, most patients with HRVC were younger than 2 years and 46% had lower respiratory tract illness, many with wheezing and bronchodilator use. The same group later published an intensive chart review of 17 patients with HRVC and found that 36% had bronchiolitis, 14% asthma, 7% COPD, and 21% persistent or hacking cough, and 3 subjects with HRVC did not have clinical data to assess. In those with bronchiolitis or asthma, no other viruses were detected.[38,59]

Lau and colleagues[36] studied 21 children with HRVC and found that wheezing or asthmatic exacerbations were common (16 of 21 oаooo, 76%), especially in those with a history of febrile wheeze or asthma. Louie and colleagues[53] studied 43 children admitted to the intensive care unit and detected HRV in 21 children. Of the 10 children in whom the virus was sequenced, 3 had HRVC; many of the patients enrolled had wheezing. Han and colleagues[54] detected HRVC in 17 Korean children hospitalized with lower respiratory tract illness, and the diagnoses were asthma exacerbation in 8 patients, bronchiolitis in 8, and pneumonia in 1. Tan and colleagues[58] reported that 2 of 64 HRV-positive specimens tested had HRVC; both these specimens were from patients with asthma and bronchiolitis. Another study determined HRVC to be associated with respiratory distress, hypoxia, and wheezing, but the numbers with HRVC were small.[48]

Four studies have not detected a clinically significant difference between HRVC and HRVA or HRVB. In a retrospective study of virus-negative bronchiolitis, Renwick and colleagues[40] found that the frequency of bronchiolitis with HRVA/HRVB (11%) was comparable to that with HRVC (12%). Similarly, Piotrowska and colleagues[51] studied

447 symptomatic children younger than 2 years and 93 asymptomatic controls and detected no associations between particular HRV genotypes and wheezing or asthma symptoms. Khetsuriani and colleagues[50] performed a case-control study of asthmatic children with acute exacerbation and those without any respiratory symptom and found both HRVA and HRVC to be significantly associated with wheezing. Calvo and colleagues[57] detected HRV in 424 of 1555 (27%) hospitalized children. The viruses from a subset of children were sequenced. There was substantial wheezing in children with HRVA and HRVC, but the investigators did not detect a difference in wheezing between children with the 2 species. Of note, 12% of healthy controls had HRV.

Several other studies have identified an association between HRVC and asthma or wheezing. Lau and colleagues[55] studied 1200 hospitalized adults and children with nasopharyngeal aspirate specimens negative for other viruses over a 1-year period and found that of the 91 HRVC-positive specimens, 78 were detected in children and 13 in adults. Of note, in this study, adults who had HRVC were more likely to present with lower respiratory tract illness than children. Nonetheless, 33 (42%) of the 78 children with HRVC infection experienced asthma exacerbations or febrile wheeze. Among the infections in adults or children, 62 (68%) occurred in patients with underlying diseases, with asthma or other chronic lung diseases being the most common. Wheezing episodes were more common in patients with HRVC (37%) and HRVA (20%) infections than in those with HRVB (0%) infection.

Taken together, these data suggest that viruses in the HRVC group may be either more prone to stimulate asthma reactivity or intrinsically more virulent. Further studies are required to determine whether these novel rhinoviruses have a greater propensity to cause exacerbation of asthma and other respiratory tract illnesses. Moreover, although the role of HRV in the ontogeny or onset of asthma is a provocative area of research,[16,32] the question of whether HRVC may drive this relationship has not been studied. The discovery of an association between disease severity or asthma risk and particular groups or strains of HRV could help inform preventive and treatment measures.

SUMMARY

It is well known that HRVs are a major trigger of asthma exacerbations in adults and children, and these viruses are now under investigation for their potential involvement in the inception of asthma. It is also clear that the newly described HRVC species account for a large proportion of HRV-related illness, including asthma and wheezing exacerbations. HRVC is genetically diverse and appears to have seasonal variations. Whether HRVC or other as yet undiscovered divergent HRV species and strains are consistently more pathogenic or asthmagenic is uncertain, and further studies are warranted.

Should an association between HRVC or certain HRV strains and more severe disease and asthma development exist, focused vaccine development targeting these strains could offer benefit for asthmatic patients of all ages. While antigenic diversity complicates passive and active prophylactic interventions (ie, antibodies or vaccines), further characterization of individual serotypes (and their neutralizing antigens) associated with severe disease could provide valuable information for developing potential preventive strategies in the future. In addition, rapid detection techniques for HRV could be used in the clinical setting to allow appropriate diagnosis and treatment of HRV-associated bronchiolitis and asthma.

ACKNOWLEDGMENTS

The author would like to thank Dr John Williams, Dr Matt Miller, Dr Natasha Halasa, and Dr Keegan Smith for critical review of the manuscript.

REFERENCES

1. Martin JA, Kochanek KD, Strobino DM, et al. Annual summary of vital statistics—2003. Pediatrics 2005;115:619–34.
2. Miller EK, Edwards KM, Weinberg GA, et al. A novel group of rhinoviruses is associated with asthma hospitalizations. J Allergy Clin Immunol 2009;123: 98–104,e1.
3. Ferreira A, Williams Z, Donninger H, et al. Rhinovirus is associated with severe asthma exacerbations and raised nasal interleukin-12. Respiration 2002;69: 136–42.
4. Gern JE. Rhinovirus respiratory infections and asthma. Am J Med 2002; 112(Suppl 6):19S–27S.
5. Hayden FG. Rhinovirus and the lower respiratory tract. Rev Med Virol 2004;14: 17–31.
6. Jartti T, Lehtinen P, Vuorinen T, et al. Respiratory picornaviruses and respiratory syncytial virus as causative agents of acute expiratory wheezing in children. Emerg Infect Dis 2004;10:1095–101.
7. Kotaniemi-Syrjanen A, Vainionpaa R, Reijonen TM, et al. Rhinovirus-induced wheezing in infancy—the first sign of childhood asthma? J Allergy Clin Immunol 2003;111:66–71.
8. Papadopoulos NG, Papi A, Psarras S, et al. Mechanisms of rhinovirus-induced asthma. Paediatr Respir Rev 2004;5:255–60.
9. Tan WC. Viruses in asthma exacerbations. Curr Opin Pulm Med 2005;11:21–6.
10. Thumerelle C, Deschildre A, Bouquillon C, et al. Role of viruses and atypical bacteria in exacerbations of asthma in hospitalized children: a prospective study in the Nord-Pas de Calais region (France). Pediatr Pulmonol 2003;35:75–82.
11. Lemanske RF Jr, Jackson DJ, Gangnon RE, et al. Rhinovirus illnesses during infancy predict subsequent childhood wheezing. J Allergy Clin Immunol 2005; 116:571–7.
12. Peltola V, Waris M, Osterback R, et al. Clinical effects of rhinovirus infections. J Clin Virol 2008;43:411–4.
13. Martinez FD, Wright AL, Taussig LM, et al. Asthma and wheezing in the first six years of life. The Group Health Medical Associates. N Engl J Med 1995;332: 133–8.
14. Miller EK, Lu X, Erdman DD, et al. Rhinovirus-associated hospitalizations in young children. J Infect Dis 2007;195:773–81.
15. Heymann PW, Carper HT, Murphy DD, et al. Viral infections in relation to age, atopy, and season of admission among children hospitalized for wheezing. J Allergy Clin Immunol 2004;114:239–47.
16. Jackson DJ, Gangnon RE, Evans MD, et al. Wheezing rhinovirus illnesses in early life predict asthma development in high-risk children. Am J Respir Crit Care Med 2008;178:667–72.
17. Pelon W, Mogabgab WJ, Phillips IA, et al. A cytopathogenic agent isolated from naval recruits with mild respiratory illnesses. Proc Soc Exp Biol Med 1957;94: 262–7.
18. Bertino JS. Cost burden of viral respiratory infections: issues for formulary decision makers. Am J Med 2002;112(Suppl 6):42S–9S.

19. Hamparian VV, Colonno RJ, Cooney MK, et al. A collaborative report: rhinoviruses—extension of the numbering system from 89 to 100. Virology 1987;159: 191–2.

20. Kaplan NM, Dove W, Abd-Eldayem SA, et al. Molecular epidemiology and disease severity of respiratory syncytial virus in relation to other potential pathogens in children hospitalized with acute respiratory infection in Jordan. J Med Virol 2008;80:168–74.

21. Kaplan NM, Dove W, Abu-Zeid AF, et al. Evidence of human metapneumovirus infection in Jordanian children. Saudi Med J 2006;27:1081–3.

22. Venarske DL, Busse WW, Griffin MR, et al. The relationship of rhinovirus-associated asthma hospitalizations with inhaled corticosteroids and smoking. J Infect Dis 2006;193:1536–43.

23. Johnston NW, Johnston SL, Norman GR, et al. The September epidemic of asthma hospitalization: school children as disease vectors. J Allergy Clin Immunol 2006;117:557–62.

24. Papadopoulos NG, Moustaki M, Tsolia M, et al. Association of rhinovirus infection with increased disease severity in acute bronchiolitis. Am J Respir Crit Care Med 2002;165:1285–9.

25. Tsolia MN, Psarras S, Bossios A, et al. Etiology of community-acquired pneumonia in hospitalized school-age children: evidence for high prevalence of viral infections. Clin Infect Dis 2004;39:681–6.

26. Blomqvist S, Roivainen M, Puhakka T, et al. Virological and serological analysis of rhinovirus infections during the first two years of life in a cohort of children. J Med Virol 2002;66:263–8.

27. Midulla F, Scagnolari C, Bonci E, et al. Respiratory syncytial virus, human bocavirus and rhinovirus bronchiolitis in infants. Arch Dis Child 2010;95:35–41.

28. Jartti T, Jartti L, Peltola V, et al. Identification of respiratory viruses in asymptomatic subjects: asymptomatic respiratory viral infections. Pediatr Infect Dis J 2008; 27:1103–7.

29. Vesa S, Kleemola M, Blomqvist S, et al. Epidemiology of documented viral respiratory infections and acute otitis media in a cohort of children followed from two to twenty-four months of age. Pediatr Infect Dis J 2001;20:574–81.

30. Johnston SL, Pattemore PK, Sanderson G, et al. The relationship between upper respiratory infections and hospital admissions for asthma: a time-trend analysis. Am J Respir Crit Care Med 1996;154:654–60.

31. Yunginger JW, Reed CE, O'Connell EJ, et al. A community-based study of the epidemiology of asthma. Incidence rates, 1964-1983. Am Rev Respir Dis 1992; 146:888–94.

32. Carroll KN, Wu P, Gebretsadik T, et al. Season of infant bronchiolitis and estimates of subsequent risk and burden of early childhood asthma. J Allergy Clin Immunol 2009;123:964–6.

33. Arden KE, McErlean P, Nissen MD, et al. Frequent detection of human rhinoviruses, paramyxoviruses, coronaviruses, and bocavirus during acute respiratory tract infections. J Med Virol 2006;78:1232–40.

34. Kistler A, Avila PC, Rouskin S, et al. Pan-viral screening of respiratory tract infections in adults with and without asthma reveals unexpected human coronavirus and human rhinovirus diversity. J Infect Dis 2007;196:817–25.

35. Lamson D, Renwick N, Kapoor V, et al. MassTag polymerase-chain-reaction detection of respiratory pathogens, including a new rhinovirus genotype, that caused influenza-like illness in New York State during 2004–2005. J Infect Dis 2006;194:1398–402.

36. Lau SK, Yip CC, Tsoi HW, et al. Clinical features and complete genome characterization of a distinct human rhinovirus (HRV) genetic cluster, probably representing a previously undetected HRV species, HRV-C, associated with acute respiratory illness in children. J Clin Microbiol 2007;45:3655–64.

37. Lee WM, Kiesner C, Pappas T, et al. A diverse group of previously unrecognized human rhinoviruses are common causes of respiratory illnesses in infants. PLoS One 2007;2:e966.

38. McErlean P, Shackelton LA, Andrews E, et al. Distinguishing molecular features and clinical characteristics of a putative new rhinovirus species, human rhinovirus C (HRV C). PLoS One 2008;3:e1847.

39. McErlean P, Shackelton LA, Lambert SB, et al. Characterisation of a newly identified human rhinovirus, HRV-QPM, discovered in infants with bronchiolitis. J Clin Virol 2007;39:67–75.

40. Renwick N, Schweiger B, Kapoor V, et al. A recently identified rhinovirus genotype is associated with severe respiratory-tract infection in children in Germany. J Infect Dis 2007;196:1754–60.

41. Palmenberg AC, Spiro D, Kuzmickas R, et al. Sequencing and analyses of all known human rhinovirus genomes reveal structure and evolution. Science 2009;324:55–9.

42. Arden KE, Mackay IM. Newly identified human rhinoviruses: molecular methods heat up the cold viruses. Rev Med Virol 2010;20:156–76.

43. Jin Y, Yuan XH, Xie ZP, et al. Prevalence and clinical characterization of a newly identified human rhinovirus C species in children with acute respiratory tract infections. J Clin Microbiol 2009;47:2895–900.

44. Huang T, Wang W, Bessaud M, et al. Evidence of recombination and genetic diversity in human rhinoviruses in children with acute respiratory infection. PLoS One 2009;4:e6355.

45. Linsuwanon P, Payungporn S, Samransamruajkit R, et al. High prevalence of human rhinovirus C infection in Thai children with acute lower respiratory tract disease. J Infect 2009;59:115–21.

46. Linsuwanon P, Payungporn S, Samransamruajkit R, et al. Recurrent human rhinovirus infections in infants with refractory wheezing. Emerg Infect Dis 2009;15: 978–80.

47. Piralla A, Rovida F, Campanini G, et al. Clinical severity and molecular typing of human rhinovirus C strains during a fall outbreak affecting hospitalized patients. J Clin Virol 2009;45:311–7.

48. Dominguez SR, Briese T, Palacios G, et al. Multiplex MassTag-PCR for respiratory pathogens in pediatric nasopharyngeal washes negative by conventional diagnostic testing shows a high prevalence of viruses belonging to a newly recognized rhinovirus clade. J Clin Virol 2008;43:219–22.

49. Briese T, Renwick N, Venter M, et al. Global distribution of novel rhinovirus genotype. Emerg Infect Dis 2008;14:944–7.

50. Khetsuriani N, Lu X, Teague WG, et al. Novel human rhinoviruses and exacerbation of asthma in children. Emerg Infect Dis 2008;14:1793–6.

51. Piotrowska Z, Vazquez M, Shapiro ED, et al. Rhinoviruses are a major cause of wheezing and hospitalization in children less than 2 years of age. Pediatr Infect Dis J 2009;28:25–9.

52. Miller EK, Khuri-Bulos N, Williams JV, et al. Human rhinovirus C associated with wheezing in hospitalised children in the Middle East. J Clin Virol 2009;46:85–9.

53. Louie JK, Roy-Burman A, Guardia-Labar L, et al. Rhinovirus associated with severe lower respiratory tract infections in children. Pediatr Infect Dis J 2009;28:337–9.

54. Han TH, Chung JY, Hwang ES, et al. Detection of human rhinovirus C in children with acute lower respiratory tract infections in South Korea. Arch Virol 2009;154: 987–91.
55. Lau SK, Yip CC, Lin AW, et al. Clinical and molecular epidemiology of human rhinovirus C in children and adults in Hong Kong reveals a possible distinct human rhinovirus C subgroup. J Infect Dis 2009;200:1096–103.
56. Wisdom A, Kutkowska AE, McWilliam Leitch EC, et al. Genetics, recombination and clinical features of human rhinovirus species C (HRV-C) infections; interactions of HRV-C with other respiratory viruses. PLoS One 2009;4:e8518.
57. Calvo C, Casas I, Garcia-Garcia ML, et al. Role of rhinovirus C respiratory infections in sick and healthy children in Spain. Pediatr Infect Dis J 2010;29(8):717–20.
58. Tan BH, Loo LH, Lim EA, et al. Human rhinovirus group C in hospitalized children, Singapore. Emerg Infect Dis 2009;15:1318–20.
59. Arden KE, Faux CE, O'Neill NT, et al. Molecular characterization and distinguishing features of a novel human rhinovirus (HRV) C, HRVC-QCE, detected in children with fever, cough and wheeze during. J Clin Virol 2003;47:219–23.

Virus/Allergen Interactions and Exacerbations of Asthma

Kirsten M. Kloepfer, MD[a,b,*], James E. Gern, MD[a,b]

KEYWORDS

• Asthma • Viral-induced wheezing • Allergic sensitization

Viral infections and allergen exposure are 2 of the most common causes of acute wheezing and exacerbations of asthma in both children and adults. Clinical research findings indicate that there are synergistic interactions between allergy and viral infection that cause increased severity of asthma exacerbations. This article summarizes the current literature linking these 2 risk factors for asthma exacerbation, and reviews experimental data suggesting potential mechanisms for interactions between viral infection and allergy that cause asthma exacerbations. Finally, the authors discuss clinical evidence that treatment of allergic inflammation could help to reduce the frequency and severity of virus-induced exacerbations of asthma.

ROLE OF VIRAL INFECTIONS IN WHEEZING ILLNESSES

Overall, 25% to 30% of infants experience at least one episode of wheezing during their first year of life. This incidence increases to 40% of children by age 3 and almost half of all children by age 6 years.[1] Two major pathogens, respiratory syncytial virus (RSV) and human rhinovirus (HRV), cause most of these illnesses. RSV is the major pathogen associated with wheezing illnesses in children younger than 2 years.[2–4] Of other viruses causing wheezing illnesses in infancy, HRV is next most common, and a variety of viruses (coronaviruses, metapneumoviruses, parainfluenza viruses, influenza viruses, bocavirus) also cause significant numbers of illnesses.

In children with established asthma, from 80% to 85% of asthma exacerbations are related to viral illness and up to two-thirds of those illnesses are caused by HRVs.[5]

---

[a] Department of Pediatrics, University of Wisconsin Madison School of Medicine and Public Health, K4/910 CSC 9988, 600 Highland Avenue, Madison, WI 53792, USA
[b] Department of Medicine, University of Wisconsin-Madison School of Medicine and Public Health, K4/910 CSC 9988, 600 Highland Avenue, Madison, WI 53792, USA
* Corresponding author. K4/910 CSC 9988, 600 Highland Avenue, Madison, WI 53792.
E-mail address: kkloepfer@medicine.wisc.edu

Immunol Allergy Clin N Am 30 (2010) 553–563
doi:10.1016/j.iac.2010.08.002
0889-8561/10/$ – see front matter © 2010 Elsevier Inc. All rights reserved.

immunology.theclinics.com

Asthma exacerbations in adults are also commonly caused by viral infections, usually HRV or influenza viruses. The etiology of virus-induced wheezing illnesses varies with the season: RSV, metapneumoviruses, and influenza viruses (with the notable exception of 2009 H1N1) are usually limited to the winter and early spring. HRV infections are most common in the spring and fall, but can occur throughout the year. Of note, asthma exacerbations are also quite seasonal, and seasonal peaks in children occur regularly in the fall and spring. In Canada, the peaks in pediatric asthma exacerbations occur approximately 17 days after Labor Day every year, and it is assumed that viral infections that are spread within schools are a major contributor to the fall peaks, and perhaps also in the spring after the children return from spring break.[6,7] It is important to bear in mind that other environmental exposures, including allergens and pollutants, also vary by season, and it seems likely that a combination of environmental factors contributes to the seasonal peaks in exacerbation rates.

ALLERGIC SENSITIZATION AS A RISK FACTOR FOR DEVELOPING VIRUS-INDUCED WHEEZE AND ASTHMA

Sensitization to aeroallergens is a risk factor for the development of asthma, particularly when it occurs in the first few years of life.[8] In addition, the prevalence of asthma is strongly related to serum IgE level.[8,9] In a recent prospective cohort study, the risk for persistent wheeze was strongly linked to early sensitization and early infection.[8] Mite-specific IgE titers of greater than 0.20 kU/L by age 2 years was associated with a 12.7% risk of persistent wheeze, increasing progressively to an 87.2% risk with increasing numbers of severe lower respiratory tract illnesses experienced.

In addition, in a longitudinal cohort, subjects with airway hyperresponsiveness (AHR) in early adulthood had higher IgE levels than subjects with past AHR or with life-long normal responsiveness.[8,10] Recent wheeze, AHR, and allergic sensitization all had a positive relation to serum IgE. The finding that young adults who are sensitized to common allergens are highly likely to have AHR even in the absence of symptoms is further evidence of the fundamental role of IgE-mediated responses in the natural history of AHR throughout childhood and into adulthood.

In a German birth cohort study, 90% of children with wheeze but no atopy lost their symptoms at school age and retained normal lung function at puberty.[11] In contrast, sensitization to perennial allergens (eg, house dust mite, cat and dog hair) developing in the first 3 years of life was associated with a loss of lung function at school age. Allergen exposure also enhanced the development of airway hyperresponsiveness in sensitized children with wheeze. Of note, sensitization and exposure later in life had much weaker relationships to airway physiology, and sensitization to seasonal allergens was not an important influence.

An Australian birth cohort study involving babies with at least one parent with allergy or asthma provides strong evidence of an interaction between allergy and viral wheeze in early life. In this study, allergic sensitization before the age of 2 years was associated with viral-induced wheezing and asthma at age 5.[12] Furthermore, there was a significant association between HRV- and RSV-induced wheezing and lower respiratory illness in the first year of life and the subsequent development of persistent wheeze at 5 years. These findings were found to be attributable only to those children who were sensitized to allergens in early life.

The Childhood Origins of Asthma (COAST) study is a high-risk birth cohort study in which families with at least one parent with allergies or asthma were enrolled prenatally, and both immune development and respiratory illnesses were prospectively evaluated.[13] Children with aeroallergen sensitization and HRV-induced wheezing during the first year of life had a high likelihood of developing asthma compared with patients with HRV wheezing within the first year of life without aeroallergen sensitization (86% vs 39%). At age 3 years, HRV wheezing status was the principal indicator of asthma risk, independent of sensitization status. Viral recovery at routine study visits was similar for children with and without asthma, suggesting that asthma is associated with greater severity of illness rather than an increased number of infections.

ALLERGY AND VIRUS-INDUCED EXACERBATIONS OF ASTHMA

There is strong clinical evidence that allergic sensitization and viral illnesses increase the risk of asthma exacerbation and hospitalization. In a cross-sectional study performed at a tertiary pediatric emergency department, allergy and viral infection (most commonly HRV) were both identified as risk factors for wheezing. Children who had HRV infection detected in combination with either eosinophilia or a positive radioallergosorbent test to common aeroallergens had the strongest odds of wheezing.[14] A second study from the same group supported these findings, and also provided evidence that many children with isolated HRV infection do not wheeze in the absence of allergic cofactors.[15] When considered together, these findings indicate that a large majority of emergent wheezing illnesses during childhood can be linked to infection with HRV, and that these wheezing attacks are most likely to occur in those who have HRV together with evidence of atopy or eosinophilic airway inflammation.

Other studies have gone one step further and have considered interactions between allergy, allergen exposure, and viral respiratory infection in causing wheezing illnesses. In a case-control study of 84 asthmatics admitted for acute exacerbations versus stable asthmatics and patients hospitalized for nonrespiratory diagnoses, a significantly higher proportion of children hospitalized for an acute exacerbation were virus-infected (44%) as compared with the stable asthmatics (18%) and nonrespiratory hospital admissions (17%; both $P<.001$).[15,16] The combination of allergic sensitization and allergen exposure was also found more frequently in asthma hospitalization group (76%) than in the 2 control groups (48% and 28%, respectively, $P<.001$). In the multivariate analysis, the viral illness and allergic sensitization/exposure were no longer significant, but the combination of these risk factors dramatically increased the risk of hospital admission (odds ratio 19.4, $P<.001$), demonstrating the link between these factors in causing asthma exacerbations. Similar findings were reported in an earlier case-control study involving adults; the combination of sensitization, high exposure to one or more indoor allergens, and viral detection considerably increased the risk of being admitted to the hospital with asthma (odds ratio 8.4, 95% confidence interval 2.1–32.8; $P = .002$).[17] Finally, in the Inner City Asthma Study (ICAS), children who were sensitized and highly exposed to cockroach allergen were more likely to be admitted to hospital, have more unscheduled medical visits, and more time off school than either nonexposed or nonsensitized children.[18] Virology was not performed in ICAS, but it can be presumed that viral infections were important contributors to asthma morbidity in this population.

Many studies have assessed the impact of allergy and viral illness on asthma exacerbations in the community. In fact, most surveillance studies have focused on detection of HRV during periods of illness, but there are limited data available regarding true rates of infection in children with asthma. It is presumed that children frequently develop asymptomatic or mild infections that do not cause asthma exacerbations. If this is true, other factors must contribute to the risk of more severe illnesses and those with wheezing. To determine the contribution of viral infections and allergic sensitization to loss of asthma control, nasal secretions were obtained weekly in a group of 58 children with asthma during peak HRV seasons (September and April).[2] As expected, virus-positive weeks were associated with greater severity of both cold and asthma symptoms. Clinically defined illnesses were then classified according to temporal association with detection of a respiratory virus. For virus-positive illnesses, the duration of cold and asthma symptoms was twice as long, and loss of asthma control occurred more frequently. Approximately two-thirds of the children were sensitized to common aeroallergens. When comparing sensitized with nonsensitized subjects, rates of infection were similar between the 2 groups; however, the sensitized group had 47% more virus-associated illnesses per season. Finally, nonsensitized subjects most commonly reported "none" or "mild" cold and asthma symptoms with their viral infections, whereas almost half of the viral infections in sensitized children resulted in moderate or severe cold or asthma symptoms (**Fig. 1**). These findings provide evidence that for children with asthma, atopy is an important risk factor for more severe cold and asthma symptoms.

RESPONSE TO EXPERIMENTAL HRV INFECTIONS IN ALLERGIC ASTHMATICS

Despite the initial assumption that HRV affects only the upper airway, studies using experimental inoculation followed by bronchoscopy or sputum induction have demonstrated HRV protein and mRNA in the lower airways.[19–21] These studies indicate that HRV infections have the potential to modify and interact with allergic airway inflammation in the lower airways. Accordingly, subjects with allergic rhinitis who were inoculated with HRV had increased levels of histamine in bronchoalveolar lavage (BAL) samples immediately and 48 hours after antigen challenge during HRV infection.[22] These same changes were not observed in nonallergic subjects infected with HRV and challenged to antigen, suggesting that the combination of viral infection and allergic disease leads to greater airway inflammation. In addition, experimentally induced HRV infection caused an enhanced eosinophilic response to allergen challenge in the allergic but not nonallergic subjects. This effect persisted for as long as 1 month after the acute HRV infection.

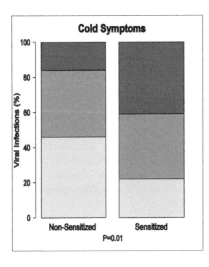
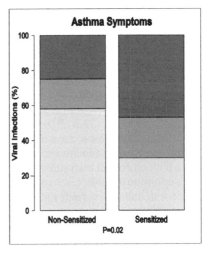
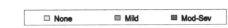

Fig. 1. Effect of sensitization on the severity of cold and asthma symptoms associated with viral infection. Mod-Sev, moderate to severe.

Two additional studies determined whether the induction of allergic inflammation would increase the severity of HRV-induced respiratory symptoms. Contrary to expectations, allergen exposure before HRV inoculation led to either no change or a slight reduction in the severity and duration of cold symptoms.[23,24] Of note is the difference in the sequence of administration of virus and allergen; this raises the question of which initiates the exacerbation, the virus or the allergic inflammation? Other factors to consider in thinking about the different outcomes of these studies are the nature of the allergen and pattern of exposure (dose and duration). It is possible that chronic low-dose allergen exposure before HRV infection amplifies the response to subsequent HRV inoculation.

Several studies have tested the theory that HRV infections cause distinct patterns of inflammation and changes in airway physiology in subjects with allergies or asthma. These studies have generally reported that the upper airway manifestations of HRV infections are similar in subjects with or without allergies or asthma, but that lower airway symptoms are increased in asthma. Two studies involving subjects with mild asthma have found similar cellular inflammation and proinflammatory cytokines in airway cells when compared with normal control subjects.[25,26] In contrast, Message and colleagues[27] found several asthma-related differences in the response to experimental HRV infection. In asthmatic subjects, HRV infection enhanced eosinophilic inflammation. In addition, virologic and clinical outcomes were related to deficient interferon (IFN)-γ and interleukin (IL)-10 responses and to augmented IL-4, IL-5, and IL-13 responses from blood and airway mononuclear cells. In a study of similar design, DeMore and colleagues[25] found that numbers of airway eosinophils preinoculation were significantly related to cold scores induced by HRV infection. Collectively, these findings suggest that eosinophilic inflammation and T-helper 2 (Th2)-biased immune responses associated with allergic sensitization enhance the clinical severity of illness associated with HRV infection.

MECHANISMS OF VIRUS-ALLERGEN INTERACTIONS

There are several potential mechanisms for allergy and viral infections to synergize in causing wheezing, airway obstruction, and exacerbations of asthma (**Box 1**). These

---

Box 1
Potential interactions between allergy and viral infections

Common underlying predisposition

- Interferon deficiency
- Th2-biased immunity
- Defect in anti-inflammatory responses

Effects of allergen-induced inflammation

- Airway hyperresponsiveness
- Mucus production
- Secondary depression of interferon synthesis

Epithelial abnormality

- Reduced barrier function
- Abnormal repair mechanisms
- Airway remodeling

mechanisms, which are not mutually exclusive, include the possibility that there are common predisposing factors, interactions related to allergic inflammation, or deficiencies in the epithelium that predispose to allergy/asthma and increased severity of viral infections.

Common Underlying Predisposition to Allergy and Viral Illnesses

Likely risk factors that would predispose to both allergy/asthma and increased severity of viral infections include genetic or acquired abnormalities that lead to either underproduction of interferons or overproduction of Th2 cytokines, leading to a Th2 bias in the immune system. Clinical studies[28,29] and experimental evidence from animal models[30] suggest that either weak T-helper 1 (Th1) responses or Th2 bias can lead to more severe viral infections, and both of these abnormalities have also been implicated as a risk factor for allergies and asthma.[31–33] In addition, children with recurrent respiratory infections were reported to have low IFN-α responses.[34] Interferons have also been related to outcomes of HRV illnesses in studies of volunteers inoculated with a safety-tested strain of HRV-16. Virus-induced IFN-γ responses in blood mononuclear cells were inversely associated with viral shedding after inoculation,[35] and stronger Th1-like responses in sputum cells (higher IFN-γ/IL-5 mRNA ratio) during induced colds were associated with milder cold symptoms and more rapid clearance of the virus.[36]

In addition to findings in the experimental inoculation model, there is evidence from clinical studies that asthma is associated with impaired virus-induced blood cell production of IFN-α and IFN-γ.[37–39] Furthermore, some studies have reported that HRV-induced epithelial cell production of IFN-β and IFN-λ is also impaired in asthma, suggesting that interferon responses in asthma are generally depressed.[40,41] On the other hand, these findings were not replicated in 2 recent studies examining cytokine responses in cultured airway epithelial cells,[42,43] and so far studies of experimentally inoculated volunteers with asthma have not found evidence of increased HRV shedding in either the upper or lower airways. Additional studies of naturally acquired colds in patients with asthma are needed to resolve these differences.

Asthma is often associated with other inflammatory diseases such as atopic dermatitis and allergic rhinitis. Together with the propensity to develop more severe illnesses with respiratory infections, these findings suggest that T-regulatory cells or other anti-inflammatory mechanisms could be impaired in asthma. To date, studies of asthma and atopic dermatitis indicate that T-regulatory cell numbers may be increased in the blood and tissues, and this paradoxic finding could represent evidence of a compensatory response to inflammation.[44,45] Important questions remain as to whether T-regulatory cell function or other anti-inflammatory regulatory mechanisms are impaired in asthma.

Finally, results obtained using animal models of respiratory viral infection suggest that biased innate immune responses to respiratory viruses in early life may establish overproduction of key cytokines such as IL-13, leading to suboptimal antiviral responses, increased risk for respiratory allergies, and changes in airway structure to promote asthma.[46] These findings suggest that early innate immune responses to viral infection could promote the development of Th2 bias, leading to allergic diseases and asthma. This concept is further supported by a recent study of gene expression patterns from peripheral blood cells of children presenting for emergency treatment of acute asthma exacerbations, mostly associated with viral respiratory infections.[47] Monocyte-dendritic cell populations had an up-regulated expression of FcϵRIα with a concomitant gene expression signature that is representative of the IL-4/IL-13-dependent "alternatively activated" phenotype. Together, these studies suggest an important link between early innate antiviral responses and the subsequent development of atopic diseases. This concept is also supported by evidence that asthma and allergy are associated with reductions in some innate antiviral responses, such as IFN-α secretion in response to Toll-like receptor (TLR)-7 and TLR-9.[48,49]

Effects of Allergen-Induced Inflammation on Antiviral Immunity

It is well established that Th1- and Th2-like responses are counterregulated, and there is recent evidence to suggest that allergic inflammation can inhibit innate immune IFN responses under some conditions. For example, engagement of IgE receptors on plasmacytoid dendritic cells leads to reduced IFN-α production in response to either TLR-9 stimulation or incubation with influenza virus.[50,51] This counterregulation between IgE-mediated and antiviral responses suggests a mechanism linking allergy, allergen exposure, and more severe viral illnesses.

There have been recent advances in understanding how environmental influences can modify dendritic cell and, subsequently, T-cell polarization through effects on the epithelium. Thymic stromal lymphopoietin (TSLP) is an epithelially derived cytokine that is induced by both viral infections and allergic inflammation. Cytokines such as IL-4 that are overproduced in asthma synergistically enhance TSLP secretion,[52] which in turn acts on dendritic cells to promote the differentiation of naïve T cells into Th2 cells. This mechanism also provides a potential mechanism for synergy between viral respiratory infections and allergic airway inflammation.

Defective Epithelial Barrier and Virus-Allergen Interactions

Viral infections damage the barrier function of the airway epithelium, and one of the consequences of this effect may be to enhance absorption of allergens and/or irritants across the airway wall, leading to an increased inflammatory response.[53] Furthermore, healthy, intact epithelial layers are difficult to infect with HRV in vitro. Viral replication is enhanced by mechanical or chemical damage to the epithelium, including removal of the apical layer of cultured epithelial cells.[54,55] These findings suggest that eosinophilic inflammation and pollutants that damage the barrier function of airway epithelium could increase susceptibility to infection and/or lead to more severe infections. This effect could be compounded in asthma because of the association between asthma and defective epithelial repair processes.[56] Finally, asthma is associated with remodeling of the airways, which includes increase in the numbers of mucus-secreting goblet cells. Experiments using epithelial cells differentiated at an air-liquid interface indicate that HRV replication is enhanced in goblet cells.[57]

DOES TREATMENT OF ALLERGIC ASTHMA DECREASE EXACERBATIONS?

Given that viral infections contribute to most exacerbations of asthma, it seems likely that effective treatment against exacerbations of asthma might also reduce the number of virus-induced exacerbations of asthma. Surprisingly, there is little or no information about the effects of asthma controllers or relievers on defined virus-induced exacerbations.

Eosinophils tend to increase during the convalescence phase following an acute upper respiratory infection in patients with allergic airway disease, and presence of eosinophils in the airways has been identified as a risk factor for more severe colds.[15,25] Furthermore, experimental HRV infection can enhance antigen-induced eosinophil influx in BAL and persistent eosinophil infiltration in bronchial mucosa and submucosa.[22,58] These findings suggest that medications that reduce eosinophil recruitment or activation might be of clinical benefit in reducing the risk of exacerbations.

Both inhaled corticosteroids and montelukast can inhibit eosinophilic airway inflammation, and reduce the risk of exacerbations (inhaled corticosteroids more so than montelukast). To date there is only indirect evidence that these treatments can specifically prevent virus-induced exacerbations.[59] A recent study showed a significant decrease in eosinophil-derived neurotoxin (EDN) levels in patients started on montelukast after an RSV infection. Furthermore, montelukast-induced reductions in EDN levels were associated with a significant decrease in wheezing episodes in follow-up.[60] Finally, omalizumab reduces the risk of exacerbations in patients with allergic asthma,[61] and provides an ideal tool to determine whether inhibiting allergic inflammation will reduce the risk for virus-induced exacerbations. Additional studies are needed to more fully explore the effects of asthma controllers on viral exacerbations.

SUMMARY

There is strong clinical evidence to support the interaction between allergy and viral infection with respect to the risk of developing asthma, and in the causation of asthma exacerbations. There is also growing evidence that asthma is associated with a defective immune response to both viruses and allergens. As we learn more about this interaction, the goal is to identify those patients who are at risk for viral-induced wheezing, treat the underlying problem, and prevent exacerbations of asthma. Understanding the mechanisms behind virus-induced asthma will help us design and use more effective treatment strategies.

REFERENCES

1. Martinez FD, Wright AL, Taussig LM, et al. Asthma and wheezing in the first six years of life. The Group Health Medical Associates. N Engl J Med 1995;332(3): 133–8.
2. Olenec JP, Kim WK, Lee WM, et al. Weekly monitoring of children with asthma for infections and illness during common cold seasons. J Allergy Clin Immunol 2010; 125(5):1001–6.
3. Sigurs N, Bjarnason R, Sigurbergsson F, et al. Respiratory syncytial virus bronchiolitis in infancy is an important risk factor for asthma and allergy at age 7. Am J Respir Crit Care Med 2000;161(5):1501–7.
4. Stein RT, Sherrill D, Morgan WJ, et al. Respiratory syncytial virus in early life and risk of wheeze and allergy by age 13 years. Lancet 1999;354(9178):541–5.
5. Johnston SL, Pattemore PK, Sanderson G, et al. Community study of role of viral infections in exacerbations of asthma in 9-11 year old children. BMJ 1995; 310(6989):1225–9.
6. Johnston NW, Johnston SL, Duncan JM, et al. The September epidemic of asthma exacerbations in children: a search for etiology. J Allergy Clin Immunol 2005;115(1):132–8.
7. Johnston NW, Johnston SL, Norman GR, et al. The September epidemic of asthma hospitalization: school children as disease vectors. J Allergy Clin Immunol 2006;117(3):557–62.
8. Holt PG, Rowe J, Kusel M, et al. Toward improved prediction of risk for atopy and asthma among preschoolers: a prospective cohort study. J Allergy Clin Immunol 2010;125(3):653–9.
9. Sears MR, Burrows B, Flannery EM, et al. Relation between airway responsiveness and serum IgE in children with asthma and in apparently normal children. N Engl J Med 1991;325(15):1067–71.

10. Peat JK, Toelle BG, Dermand J, et al. Serum IgE levels, atopy, and asthma in young adults: results from a longitudinal cohort study. Allergy 1996;51(11):804–10.

11. Illi S, von ME, Lau S, et al. Perennial allergen sensitisation early in life and chronic asthma in children: a birth cohort study. Lancet 2006;368(9537):763–70.

12. Kusel MM, de Klerk NH, Kebadze T, et al. Early-life respiratory viral infections, atopic sensitization, and risk of subsequent development of persistent asthma. J Allergy Clin Immunol 2007;119(5):1105–10.

13. Jackson DJ, Gangnon RE, Evans MD, et al. Wheezing rhinovirus illnesses in early life predict asthma development in high-risk children. Am J Respir Crit Care Med 2008;178(7):667–72.

14. Duff AL, Pomeranz ES, Gelber LE, et al. Risk factors for acute wheezing in infants and children: viruses, passive smoke, and IgE antibodies to inhalant allergens. Pediatrics 1993;92(4):535–40.

15. Rakes GP, Arruda E, Ingram JM, et al. Rhinovirus and respiratory syncytial virus in wheezing children requiring emergency care. IgE and eosinophil analyses. Am J Respir Crit Care Med 1999;159(3):785–90.

16. Murray CS, Poletti G, Kebadze T, et al. Study of modifiable risk factors for asthma exacerbations: virus infection and allergen exposure increase the risk of asthma hospital admissions in children. Thorax 2006;61(5):376–82.

17. Green RM, Custovic A, Sanderson G, et al. Synergism between allergens and viruses and risk of hospital admission with asthma: case-control study. BMJ 2002;324(7340):763.

18. Rosenstreich DL, Eggleston P, Kattan M, et al. The role of cockroach allergy and exposure to cockroach allergen in causing morbidity among inner-city children with asthma. N Engl J Med 1997;336(19):1356–63.

19. Gern JE, Calhoun W, Swenson C, et al. Rhinovirus infection preferentially increases lower airway responsiveness in allergic subjects. Am J Respir Crit Care Med 1997;155(6):1872–6.

20. Mosser AG, Vrtis R, Burchell L, et al. Quantitative and qualitative analysis of rhinovirus infection in bronchial tissues. Am J Respir Crit Care Med 2005;171(6):645–51.

21. Papadopoulos NG, Bates PJ, Bardin PG, et al. Rhinoviruses infect the lower airways. J Infect Dis 2000;181(6):1875–84.

22. Calhoun WJ, Dick EC, Schwartz LB, et al. A common cold virus, rhinovirus 16, potentiates airway inflammation after segmental antigen bronchoprovocation in allergic subjects. J Clin Invest 1994;94:2200–8.

23. Avila PC, Abisheganaden JA, Wong H, et al. Effects of allergic inflammation of the nasal mucosa on the severity of rhinovirus 16 cold. J Allergy Clin Immunol 2000; 105(5):923–32.

24. De Kluijver J, Evertse CE, Sont JK, et al. Are rhinovirus-induced airway responses in asthma aggravated by chronic allergen exposure? Am J Respir Crit Care Med 2003;168:1174–80.

25. DeMore JP, Weisshaar EH, Vrtis RF, et al. Similar colds in subjects with allergic asthma and nonatopic subjects after inoculation with rhinovirus-16. J Allergy Clin Immunol 2009;124(2):245–52.

26. Fleming HE, Little FF, Schnurr D, et al. Rhinovirus-16 colds in healthy and in asthmatic subjects: similar changes in upper and lower airways. Am J Respir Crit Care Med 1999;160(1):100–8.

27. Message SD, Laza-Stanca V, Mallia P, et al. Rhinovirus-induced lower respiratory illness is increased in asthma and related to virus load and Th1/2 cytokine and IL-10 production. Proc Natl Acad Sci U S A 2008;105(36):13562–7.

28. Copenhaver CC, Gern JE, Li Z, et al. Cytokine response patterns, exposure to viruses, and respiratory infections in the first year of life. Am J Respir Crit Care Med 2004;170:175–80.
29. Gern JE, Brooks GD, Meyer P, et al. Bidirectional interactions between viral respiratory illnesses and cytokine responses in the first year of life. J Allergy Clin Immunol 2006;117:72–8.
30. Rosenthal LA, Mikus LD, Tuffaha A, et al. Attenuated innate mechanisms of interferon-gamma production in rats susceptible to postviral airway dysfunction. Am J Respir Cell Mol Biol 2004;30(5):702–9.
31. Heaton T, Rowe J, Turner S, et al. An immunoepidemiological approach to asthma: identification of in-vitro T-cell response patterns associated with different wheezing phenotypes in children. Lancet 2005;365(9454):142–9.
32. Holt PG, Upham JW, Sly PD. Contemporaneous maturation of immunologic and respiratory functions during early childhood: implications for development of asthma prevention strategies. J Allergy Clin Immunol 2005;116(1):16–24.
33. Stern DA, Guerra S, Halonen M, et al. Low IFN-gamma production in the first year of life as a predictor of wheeze during childhood. J Allergy Clin Immunol 2007; 120(4):835–41.
34. Isaacs D, Clarke JR, Tyrrell DA, et al. Deficient production of leucocyte interferon (interferon-alpha) in vitro and in vivo in children with recurrent respiratory tract infections. Lancet 1981;2(8253):950–2.
35. Parry DE, Busse WW, Sukow KA, et al. Rhinovirus-induced peripheral blood mononuclear cell responses and outcome of experimental infection in allergic subjects. J Allergy Clin Immunol 2000;105:692–8.
36. Gern JE, Vrtis R, Grindle KA, et al. Relationship of upper and lower airway cytokines to outcome of experimental rhinovirus infection. Am J Respir Crit Care Med 2000;162:2226–31.
37. Bufe A, Gehlhar K, Grage-Griebenow E, et al. Atopic phenotype in children is associated with decreased virus-induced interferon-alpha release. Int Arch Allergy Immunol 2002;127(1):82–8.
38. Gehlhar K, Bilitewski C, Reinitz-Rademacher K, et al. Impaired virus-induced interferon-alpha2 release in adult asthmatic patients. Clin Exp Allergy 2006; 36(3):331–7.
39. Papadopoulos NG, Stanciu LA, Papi A, et al. Rhinovirus-induced alterations on peripheral blood mononuclear cell phenotype and costimulatory molecule expression in normal and atopic asthmatic subjects. Clin Exp Allergy 2002; 32(4):537–42.
40. Contoli M, Message SD, Laza-Stanca V, et al. Role of deficient type III interferon-lambda production in asthma exacerbations. Nat Med 2006;12(9):1023–6.
41. Wark PA, Johnston SL, Bucchieri F, et al. Asthmatic bronchial epithelial cells have a deficient innate immune response to infection with rhinovirus. J Exp Med 2005; 201(6):937–47.
42. Bochkov YA, Hanson KM, Keles S, et al. Rhinovirus-induced modulation of gene expression in bronchial epithelial cells from subjects with asthma. Mucosal Immunol 2010;3:69–80.
43. Lopez-Souza N, Favoreto S, Wong H, et al. In vitro susceptibility to rhinovirus infection is greater for bronchial than for nasal airway epithelial cells in human subjects. J Allergy Clin Immunol 2009;123(6):1384–90.
44. Caproni M, Antiga E, Torchia D, et al. FoxP3-expressing T regulatory cells in atopic dermatitis lesions. Allergy Asthma Proc 2007;28(5):525–8.

45. Smyth LJ, Eustace A, Kolsum U, et al. Increased airway T regulatory cells in asthmatic subjects. Chest 2010. [Epub ahead of print]. DOI:10.1378/chest.09-3079.

46. Benoit LA, Holtzman MJ. New immune pathways from chronic post-viral lung disease. Ann N Y Acad Sci 2010;1183:195–210.

47. Subrata LS, Bizzintino J, Mamessier E, et al. Interactions between innate antiviral and atopic immunoinflammatory pathways precipitate and sustain asthma exacerbations in children. J Immunol 2009;183(4):2793–800.

48. Roponen M, Yerkovich ST, Hollams E, et al. Toll-like receptor 7 function is reduced in adolescents with asthma. Eur Respir J 2010;35(1):64–71.

49. Tversky JR, Le TV, Bieneman AP, et al. Human blood dendritic cells from allergic subjects have impaired capacity to produce interferon-alpha via Toll-like receptor 9. Clin Exp Allergy 2008;38(5):781–8.

50. Gill MA, Bajwa G, George TA, et al. Counterregulation between the FcepsilonRI pathway and antiviral responses in human plasmacytoid dendritic cells. J Immunol 2010;184(11):5999–6006.

51. Schroeder JT, Bieneman AP, Xiao H, et al. TLR9- and FcepsilonRI-mediated responses oppose one another in plasmacytoid dendritic cells by down-regulating receptor expression. J Immunol 2005;175(9):5724–31.

52. Kato A, Favoreto S Jr, Avila PC, et al. TLR3- and Th2 cytokine-dependent production of thymic stromal lymphopoietin in human airway epithelial cells. J Immunol 2007;179(2):1080–7.

53. Sakamoto M, Ida S, Takishima T. Effect of influenza virus infection on allergic sensitization to aerosolized ovalbumin in mice. J Immunol 1984; 132:2614–7.

54. Jakiela B, Brockman-Schneider R, Amineva S, et al. Basal cells of differentiated bronchial epithelium are more susceptible to rhinovirus infection. Am J Respir Cell Mol Biol 2008;38(5):517–23.

55. Lopez-Souza N, Dolganov G, Dubin R, et al. Resistance of differentiated human airway epithelium to infection by rhinovirus. Am J Physiol Lung Cell Mol Physiol 2004;286(2):L373–81.

56. Holgate ST, Roberts G, Arshad HS, et al. The role of the airway epithelium and its interaction with environmental factors in asthma pathogenesis. Proc Am Thorac Soc 2009;6(8):655–9.

57. Lachowicz-Scroggins ME, Boushey HA, Finkbeiner WE, et al. Interleukin-13 induced mucous metaplasia increases susceptibility of human airway epithelium to rhinovirus infection. Am J Respir Cell Mol Biol 2010. [Epub ahead of print]. DOI:10.1165/rcmb.2000 0244OC.

58. Lemanske RF Jr, Dick EC, Swenson CA, et al. Rhinovirus upper respiratory infection increases airway hyperreactivity and late asthmatic reactions. J Clin Invest 1989;83(1):1–10.

59. Johnston NW, Mandhane PJ, Dai J, et al. Attenuation of the September epidemic of asthma exacerbations in children: a randomized, controlled trial of montelukast added to usual therapy. Pediatrics 2007;120(3):e702–12.

60. Kim CK, Choi J, Kim HB, et al. A randomized intervention of montelukast for post-bronchiolitis: effect on eosinophil degranulation. J Pediatr 2010;156(5): 749–54.

61. Busse WW, Massanari M, Kianifard F, et al. Effect of omalizumab on the need for rescue systemic corticosteroid treatment in patients with moderate-to-severe persistent IgE-mediated allergic asthma: a pooled analysis. Curr Med Res Opin 2007;23(10):2379–86.

Bacterial Infections and Pediatric Asthma

Matti Korppi, MD, PhD

KEYWORDS

- Asthma • Child • Pneumococcus • Mycoplasma
- Chlamydophila

In the first half of the the 20th century, asthma was considered to be precipitated and prolonged by bacterial infections, and several bacteria, including *Streptococcus pneumoniae* and *Haemophilus influenzae,* were considered to have a central role in asthma.[1] Investigators suggested that bacterial allergy or chronic focal infections, like sinusitis or adenoiditis, could be the cause of asthma.[2] In the second half of the 20th century, the connection between asthma and viruses was revealed in both epidemiologic and clinical studies.[3] Currently, most wheezing episodes and asthma exacerbations in children are known to be precipitated by viruses and respiratory syncytial virus (RSV), rhinovirus and bocavirus seem to have a special role.[3,4] Whether viruses attend the emergence of asthma, or only trigger symptoms in susceptible individuals, has thus far remained unresolved. Concomitantly with studies on viruses and asthma, some evidence has been found to relate infections with atypical bacteria *Mycoplasma pneumoniae* and *Chlamydophila pneumoniae* with asthma exacerbations and asthma severity.[5] However, clinical trials involving antibiotics effective against *M pneumoniae* and *C pneumoniae*, as well as antibiotics and surgical treatments for sinusitis and adenoiditis, have failed to demonstrate any sustained clinical benefits.[1,2]

The aim of the present review was to evaluate the currently available data on the role of bacterial infections in pediatric asthma, with a special focus on early-life colonization, involvement by atypical bacteria and use of antibiotics.

ASTHMA PHENOTYPES IN CHILDREN

A third of all children suffer from infection-induced wheezing during the first 3 years of life,[6,7] and in 1%–3% of cases, symptoms are severe enough to need hospital care.[7] About 60% of early childhood wheezers have transient wheezing with symptoms only during respiratory infections at less than 3 years of age.[6,8] In them, lung function may

No funding support.
No financial disclosure.
Pediatric Research Center, Tampere University and University Hospital, Finmed-3 building, Tampere University 33014, Finland
E-mail address: matti.korppi@uta.fi

be subnormal before any infection or wheezing takes place, and improves by time though does not catch-up healthy subjects during childhood.[8,9]

About 40% of early childhood wheezers have persistent wheezing from 3 to 6 years of age. Half of them become sensitized to inhaled allergens before school age, which means a significant risk of chronic asthma at school age.[7,10] In typical cases, wheezing episodes start during the second or third year of life, are induced by rhinoviruses[11] and are associated with increased airway reactivity throughout childhood.[6,8]

In contrast, persistent wheezers with no allergic sensitization usually start wheezing before one year of age, typically induced by RSV infection.[12] They subsequently wheeze mainly during respiratory infections, with a decreasing tendency with age.[6,13] At the age of 13 years, the risk for wheezing is only slightly increased, whereas lung function remains subnormal through childhood, including also non-symptomatic cases.[6,8]

Thus, the majority of children with wheezing and asthma outgrow their symptoms by school age, but based on recent long-term follow-up studies, asthma relapses and subnormal lung function are common in young adults.[14–17] These studies have highlighted parental asthma, maternal smoking and wheezing induced by viruses other than RSV as predictive factors for later asthma.[14,15]

BACTERIAL COLONIZATION IN INFANCY AND ASTHMA IN CHILDHOOD

The hygiene hypothesis was proposed some twenty years ago and has been widely used as a frame of references in asthma and allergy studies.[18] According to the hypothesis, a lack of early childhood exposure to beneficial infectious agents, like probiotics and other symbiotic bacteria of the gut flora increases susceptibility to allergic diseases by modulating the maturing immune system in the direction of T helper cell 2 (Th2)-mediated immunity. Many bacteria and viruses elicit a Th1-mediated immune response, which downregulates Th2 responses.[19] Thus, an insufficient stimulation of the Th1 arm of the immune system may lead to an overactive Th2 arm. A more sophisticated explanation is that the exposure to beneficial microbes in urban conditions remains insufficient for the development of regulatory T cells to balance the Th1 and Th2 responses.[20]

While the hygiene hypothesis stresses the beneficial role of symbiotic intestinal bacteria, the early-life colonization with certain other strains like respiratory pathogens may be harmful (**Table 1**). Benn and colleagues[21] cultured vaginal samples for bacteria from around 3000 Danish women during pregnancy, and followed-up their children until five years of age. Early wheezing, assessed as hospitalization for asthma or wheezing at 0–3 years of age, was associated with maternal vaginal colonization with *Ureaplasma urealyticum* during pregnancy.[21] Childhood asthma, assessed as the use of medication for asthma between 4 and 5 years of age, was associated with vaginal colonization with *Staphylococcus aureus* and maternal use of antibiotics during pregnancy. In adjusted analyses, both *S aureus* colonization and maternal antibiotic use were independently significant risk factors for asthma.[21] Thus, the composition of maternal micro-flora during pregnancy may be associated with the risk of wheezing and asthma in the offspring, and early-life wheezing and childhood asthma seem to have different microbial risk factors.

Bisgaard and colleagues[22] followed a birth cohort of children born to mothers with asthma until the age of 5 years. Hypopharyngeal aspirates from 321 neonates at one month of age were cultured for bacteria and 21% were colonized with *S pneumoniae*, *M catarrhalis* or *H influenzae*. This colonization was associated with subsequent wheezing, including hospitalizations for wheezing, but colonization with *S aureus* was not.[22] Further, this colonization with respiratory pathogens was associated with

Table 1
Prenatal and postnatal exposure to bacteria and antibiotics as risk factors of later asthma

Microbe/Antibiotics	Colonization/Exposure to Antibiotics	Outcomes	References
Streptococcus pneumoniae, non-typeable *Haemophilus influenzae, Moraxella catarrhalis*	Colonization at <4 weeks of age	Increased asthma risk at 5 years of age	Bisgaard et al[22]
Staphylococcus aureus	Maternal colonization during pregnancy	Increased asthma risk at 5 years of age	Benn et al[21]
Antibiotic therapy	Maternal use during pregnancy	Increased asthma risk at 5 years of age	Benn et al[21]
Antibiotic therapy	Children at age <1 month	Wheezing at age <12 months	Alm et al[28]
Antibiotic therapy	Children at age <3 months	Wheezing at age 1.5 years	Wickens et al[27]
Antibiotic therapy	Children at <12 months of age	Increased asthma risk at 6–7 years of age	Kozyrskyj et al[24] Foliaki et al[25]

doctor-diagnosed asthma (33% vs 10%) and reversibility of airway resistance (23% vs 18%) at age five years.[22] Instead, bacterial colonization at one year of age was not a predictor of subsequent wheezing or asthma, which stresses the importance of the events during the first weeks of life.[22] There is no straightforward explanation for the results. Early-life bacterial colonization may induce prolonged neutrophilic inflammation of the airways, which is characteristic of non-atopic infection-induced asthma; or bacterial colonization may only indicate a defective immunity presenting in early life in children susceptible to asthma. Despite the mechanism, the results confirm that early-life colonization with bacterial pathogens is not beneficial (see **Table 1**).

ANTIBIOTICS IN EARLY LIFE AS RISK FACTORS FOR ASTHMA

Many retrospective surveys and some health care database studies have revealed that the use of antibiotics in early life is a risk factor for later asthma (see **Table 1**), as summarized by Marra and colleagues[23] in their meta-analysis and systematic review. Six birth cohort studies have been published after this meta-analysis.[24-29] In the birth cohorts from the U.S.[24] and Europe,[25] the use of antibiotics during the first year of life was an independent risk factor for asthma at 6–7 years of age. On the other hand, no association was found between the use of antibiotics in early life and asthma at five years of age in an Australian cohort.[26] Wickens and colleagues[27] collected data on antibiotic exposure before 3 months of age and asthma diagnoses at 1.5, 3 and 4 years of age. This early exposure to antibiotics was associated with asthma at 1.5 years of age, but the finding was not robust to adjustment for respiratory infections at the same age. No association was found with asthma at 3 or 4 years of age. Similarly, neonatal antibiotic use was a risk factor for early childhood wheezing in a Swedish birth cohort.[28] Marra and colleagues[29] combined data on more than 250,000 children from seven birth cohorts, and exposure to antibiotics before 12 months of age was associated with an increased asthma risk at 2–9 years of age. The hazard rate was significant but rather low, 1.12 to 1.17, in the adjusted analyses and supplementary sensitivity analyses. The increased risk was equal for all antibiotics. The increasing number of courses was associated with an increasing asthma risk suggesting a dose-response relationship.[29] Thus, the recent prospective population-based studies have confirmed the association between antibiotic exposure in infancy and later asthma, but the risk of asthma is rather small.

STREPTOCOCCUS PNEUMONIAE, HAEMOPHILUS INFLUENZAE AND MORAXELLA CATARRHALIS

S pneumoniae, noncapsulated H influenzae and M catarrhalis are common inhabitants of the upper respiratory tract of children, but they seem to play no or only minor role in asthma exacerbations. In agreement with this idea, 34.2% of children with recurrent wheezing, 43.4% of those with acute wheezing and 39.3% of those with no wheezing were colonized by respiratory pathogens in a recent ten-year study consisting of 1200 asthma treatment episodes from Japan.[30] On the other hand, serologic evidence of bacterial infection was found in 21% of 188 wheezing children less than six years of age[31] and in 18% of 220 wheezing children aged 3 to 16 years.[32] In these two Finnish studies, 45% of the involvements were pneumococcal, and when PCR for rhino- and enteroviruses was available, two-thirds of the pneumococcal findings were mixed cases with picornaviruses.[32]

Pneumococcus causes a third of pneumonia cases at all ages.[33] Clinical experience suggests that asthma treatment balance worsens during pneumonia, but no evidence is available that S pneumoniae had any specific role in asthma exacerbations. Adults who have asthma seem to have an increased risk of invasive pneumococcal infections.[34] Non-capsulated H influenzae is an important trigger of the exacerbations of chronic obstructive pulmonary disease in adults. An antibody response to H influenzae was demonstrated in 2%–8% of wheezing children, usually with a simultaneous response to viruses.[31,32] The occasional M catarrhalis findings in wheezing children have all been co-infections with virus.[31,32] In children, frequent pneumococcal and other bacterial airway infections lead to wet cough, protracted bronchitis and suppurating lung disease rather than to asthma and these other conditions are easily misdiagnosed as asthma.[35,36]

MYCOPLASMA PNEUMONIAE, CHLAMYDOPHILA PNEUMONIAE AND CHLAMYDIA SPECIES

M pneumoniae may induce wheezing and asthma symptoms in children,[37–42] but there is no substantial evidence of an active role of Mycoplasma infection in the pathogenesis or inception of chronic asthma (**Table 2**). The presence of antibodies to M pneumoniae in children with asthma was associated with subsequent asthma exacerbations, but the finding has not been confirmed.[40] In a recent study of 65 children less than five years of age, M pneumoniae infection was not associated with asthma, bronchial hyper-responsiveness or lung function abnormalities two years later.[43]

The identification rates for Chlamydophila strains have varied from 4% to 25% in children with asthma exacerbation.[37–39,42,43] Acute episodes of C pneumoniae infections may be primary infections or reactivations of chronic infections, probably induced by acute viral infections.[44] C pneumoniae may cause an occult chronic infection and inflammation in the airways, and thus participate in the inception or pathogenesis of asthma (see **Table 2**). In line with this, viable Chlamydophila organisms were detected by culture in a third of bronchoalveolar lavage samples obtained from 42 children with treatment-resistant asthma.[45] On the other hand, no differences were observed in antibodies to C pneumoniae in population-based case-control studies

Table 2
The role of atypical bacteria in asthma exacerbation, in chronic stable asthma and in the onset of new asthma in children

Microbe	Asthma Exacerbation	Stable Asthma	Incipient Asthma	References
Mycoplasma pneumoniae	Yes	No	No	37–42
Chlamydophila pneumoniae	Yes	Yes	Yes?	37–39,42,43,45,48,49
Chlamydia trachomatis	Yes?	Yes?	No?	48

in children and young adults with asthma[46] and in children less than six years old with incipient asthma.[47]

Recently, Webley and colleagues[48] performed bronchoscopy and obtained lung lavage fluid samples from 182 children with treatment-resistant chronic lung disease. *Chlamydophila* or *Chlamydia* species were detected by PCR in 124 (68%) children; 43% were positive for *C pneumoniae*, 42% for *C trachomatis* and 26% for both. The positivity to *C trachomatis* decreased and to *C pneumoniae* increased with age. Fifty-nine (46%) of the 128 asthma patients were culture-positive for *Chlamydophila*. The authors concluded that viable *C trachomatis* and *C pneumoniae* occur more frequently than previously believed in children with treatment-resistant asthma.[48] Ten years ago, Cunningham and colleagues[49] detected *C pneumoniae* by PCR in nasal washes in 23% of children with asthma exacerbation. Though the presence of *C pneumoniae* was not predictive of subsequent symptoms, the duration of PCR positivity and the presence of *Chlamydophila*-specific secretory IgA were associated with the number of exacerbations during the 12-month follow-up period. These observations highlight the role of *Chlamydophila* species in asthma in children, and the role of *C trachomatis* needs to be further evaluated (see **Table 2**).

ANTIBIOTIC TREATMENT FOR ACUTE AND CHRONIC ASTHMA

Bacterial infections in children with asthma, including children with an acute asthma exacerbation, should be treated according to the general principles of antibiotic therapy, as described in a recent review.[3] In clinical practice, however, antibiotics are prescribed more frequently for respiratory tract infection if the children have asthma compared with non-asthmatic children.[50,51] Data from adults suggest that patients with an asthma exacerbation may benefit from treatment with macrolides, ketolides, tetracyclines or fluoroquinolones.[52,53] Five studies including 357 adults with asthma were accepted in a systematic review,[54] and macrolides had a beneficial effect on symptoms and eosinophilic markers of inflammation, but only in patients with serologic evidence of *Chlamydophila* infection **Table 3**.

There have been only two pediatric studies on asthma treatment by antibiotics, and both offered some evidence for the efficacy of macrolides that might be worth studying further. Strunk and colleagues[55] determined the budesonide and salmeterol dose needed to control symptoms in 292 children more than 6 years old with moderate-to-severe asthma. Thereafter, montelukast, azithromycin or placebo was administered randomly to 55 children. The primary outcome was the time from randomization to inadequate asthma control. The median time in the azithromycin

Table 3		
Asthma Course	**Antibiotics for Typical Bacteria**	**Antibiotics for Atypical Bacteria**
	Streptococcus pneumonia *Haemophilus influenzae* *Moraxella catarrhalis*	*Mycoplasma pneumoniae* *Chlamydophila pneumoniae* *Chlamydia trachomatis*
Asthma exacerbation	No	Yes, if microbiologically identified or clinically strongly suspected
Stable asthma	No	No
Incipient asthma	No	No

group was 8.4 weeks, compared with 13.9 weeks in the montelukast group and 19.1 weeks in the placebo group. The result was not statistically significant but strongly suggested that azithromycin was not a clinically effective corticosteroid-sparing alternative in children with asthma. Esposito and colleagues[56] studied 352 children aged one to four years with recurrent lower respiratory tract infections, including also wheezing children. Patients were randomized to receive either azithromycin and bronchodilators, or bronchodilators alone for three weeks. Macrolide therapy significantly decreased the symptoms, but only for the first month, and only in children with serologic and/or PCR evidence of *Chlamydophila* infection.

FUTURE PERSPECTIVES

The application of molecular methods started a new era in the study of respiratory viruses in the pathogenesis of asthma. The studies have changed our concept about the role of the 'old' viruses, such as rhino- and enteroviruses, and helped to find new important viruses, such as bocavirus.[3,4] Only about one percent of all bacteria can be cultured in the laboratory, and recent studies using sensitive molecular methods have shown that the microbiota of humans is much more varied than earlier believed.[57] In 2010, Hilty and colleagues[58] published their results on the bacterial flora of lower airways assessed by molecular methods, and they concluded that the bronchial tree is not sterile but contains a characteristic microbial flora. The microbial flora is rather similar in adults and children but differs between healthy individuals and those with disease. Anaerobic bacteria were the major colonizing strains in controls, whereas Proteobacteria including well-known pathogens *Haemophilus, Moraxella* and *Neisseria* species were the predominant bacteria in children with asthma. In addition, *Staphylococcus* and *Streptococcus* species were also present in excess in children with asthma. The results provide strong though preliminary evidence that lower airways have a characteristic normal microbiota, which consists of protective bacteria and that the composition of this population can be disturbed in lung diseases like asthma. Whether pathogens in asthmatic airways are secondary to mucosal damage or capable of inducing or maintaining chronic airway inflammation, remains to be seen in further studies.

If children with asthma have disturbed bacterial flora in the airways, the crucial question is: how can the protective flora be restored and maintained. Obviously, antibiotics are not the solution to this problem. Instead, the availability of vaccines that are effective not only against *S pneumoniae* but also non-capsulated *H influenzae* opens new possibilities for large-scale interventions.

SUMMARY

Typical bacteria, like *S pneumoniae*, *H influenzae*, *M catarrhalis* and *S aureus,* seem to have no role in asthma in children. Atypical bacteria, like *M pneumoniae*,

C pneumoniae and probably also *C trachomatis* can induce wheezing and cause asthma exacerbations in children, and chronic *Chlamydophila* infections may even participate in asthma pathogenesis. However, studies have failed to show any benefits from antibiotics in preventing incipient or stable pediatric asthma. In line with this, the evidence for the use of antibiotics effective against atypical bacteria in asthma exacerbations in children is marginal. Exposure to antibiotics in utero and in infancy has been an independent risk factor for later asthma in many studies; in some cases even demonstrating a dose-response relationship. A recent study using sensitive molecular biology methods to analyze samples from the lower airways provided preliminary evidence that lower airways are not sterile but have their own protective microbiota which can be disturbed in lung diseases like asthma.

REFERENCES

1. Black PN. Antibiotics for the treatment of asthma. Curr Opin Pharmacol 2007;7: 266–71.
2. Korppi M. Management of bacterial infections in children with asthma. Expert Rev Anti Infect Ther 2009;7:869–77.
3. Papadopoulos NG, Kalobatsou A. Respiratory viruses in childhood asthma. Curr Opin Allergy Clin Immunol 2007;7:91–5.
4. Allander T, Jartti T, Gupta S, et al. Human bocavirus and acute wheezing in children. Clin Infect Dis 2007;44:904–10.
5. Esposito S, Principi N. Asthma in children: are chlamydia or mycoplasma involved? Paediatr Drugs 2001;3:159–68.
6. Taussig LM, Wright AL, Holberg CJ, et al. Tucson children's respiratory study: 1980 to present. J Allergy Clin Immunol 2003;111:661–75.
7. Piippo-Savolainen E, Korppi M. Long-term outcomes of early childhood wheezing. Curr Opin Allergy Clin Immunol 2009;9:190–6.
8. Morgan WJ, Stern DA, Sherrill DL, et al. Outcome of asthma and wheezing in the first 6 years of life: follow-up through adolescence. Am J Respir Crit Care Med 2005;172:1253–8.
9. Turner SW, Young S, Landau LI, et al. Reduced lung function both before bronchiolitis and at 11 years. Arch Dis Child 2002;87:417–20.
10. Sherrill D, Stein R, Kurzius-Spencer M, et al. On early sensitization to allergens and development of respiratory symptoms. Clin Exp Allergy 1999;29:905–11.
11. Kotaniemi-Syrjänen A, Vainionpää R, Reijonen TM, et al. Rhinovirus-induced wheezing in infancy - the first sign of childhood asthma? J Allergy Clin Immunol 2003;111:66–71.
12. Stein RT, Sherrill D, Morgan WJ, et al. Respiratory syncytial virus in early life and risk of wheeze and allergy by age 13 years. Lancet 1999;354:541–5.
13. Halonen M, Stern DA, Lohman IC, et al. Two subphenotypes of childhood asthma that differ in maternal and paternal influences and asthma risk. Am J Respir Crit Care Med 1999;160:564–70.
14. Piippo-Savolainen E, Remes S, Kannisto S, et al. Asthma and lung function 20 years after wheezing in infancy. Results from a prospective follow-up. Arch Pediatr Adolesc Med 2004;158:1070–6.
15. Goksör E, Åmark M, Alm B, et al. Asthma symptoms in early childhood- what happens then? Acta Paediatr 2006;95:471–8.
16. Stern DA, Morgan WJ, Halonen M, et al. Wheezing and bronchial hyper-responsiveness in early childhood as predictors of newly diagnosed asthma in early adulthood: a longitudinal birth-cohort study. Lancet 2008;372:1058–64.

17. Stern DA, Morgan WJ, Wright AL, et al. Poor airway function in early infancy and lung function by age 22 years: a non-selective longitudinal cohort study. Lancet 2007;370:758–64.
18. Strachan DP. Family size, infection and atopy: the first decade of the "hygiene hypothesis". Thorax 2000;55(Suppl 1):S2–10.
19. Folkerts G, Walzl G, Openshaw PJ. Do common childhood infections 'teach' the immune system not to be allergic? Immunol Today 2000;21:118–20.
20. Bufford JD, Gern JE. The hygiene hypothesis revisited. Immunol Allergy Clin North Am 2005;25:247–62.
21. Benn CS, Thorsen P, Jensen JS, et al. Maternal vaginal microflora during pregnancy and the risk of asthma hospitalization and use of antiasthma medication in early childhood. J Allergy Clin Immunol 2002;110:72–7.
22. Bisgaard H, Hermansen MN, Buchvald F, et al. Childhood asthma after bacterial colonization of the airway in neonates. N Engl J Med 2007;357:1487–95.
23. Marra F, Lynd L, Coombes M, et al. Does antibiotic exposure during infancy lead to development of asthma? a systematic review and meta-analysis. Chest 2006;129:610–8.
24. Kozyrskyj AL, Ernst P, Becker AB. Increased risk of childhood asthma from antibiotic use in early life. Chest 2007;131:1753–9.
25. Foliaki S, Foliaki S, Pearce N, et al. Antibiotic use in infancy and symptoms of asthma, rhinoconjunctivitis, and eczema in children 6 and 7 years old: international study of asthma and allergies in childhood phase III. J Allergy Clin Immunol 2009;124:982–9.
26. Kusel MM, de Klerk N, Holt PG, et al. Antibiotic use in the first year of life and risk of atopic disease in early childhood. Clin Exp Allergy 2008;38:1921–8.
27. Wickens K, Ingham T, Epton M, et al. The association of early life exposure to antibiotics and the development of asthma, eczema and atopy in a birth cohort: confounding or causality? Clin Exp Allergy 2008;38:1318–24.
28. Alm B, Erdes L, Möllborg P, et al. Neonatal antibiotic treatment is a risk factor for early wheezing. Pediatrics 2008;12:697–702.
29. Marra F, Marra CA, Richardson K, et al. Antibiotic use in children is associated with increased risk of asthma. Pediatrics 2009;123:1003–10.
30. Nagayama Y, Tsubaki T, Nakayama S, et al. Bacterial colonization in respiratory secretions from acute and recurrent wheezing infants and children. Pediatr Allergy Immunol 2007;18:110–7.
31. Korppi M, Leinonen M, Koskela M, et al. Bacterial infection in under school age children with expiratory difficulty. Pediatr Pulmonol 1991;10:254–9.
32. Lehtinen P, Jartti T, Virkki R, et al. Bacterial coinfections in children with viral wheezing. Eur J Clin Microbiol Infect Dis 2006;25:463–9.
33. Heiskanen-Kosma T, Korppi M, Jokinen C, et al. Etiology of childhood pneumonia: serologic results of a prospective, population-based study. Pediatr Infect Dis J 1998;17:986–91.
34. Talbot TR, Hartert TV, Mitchel E, et al. Asthma as a risk factor for invasive pneumococcal disease. N Engl J Med 2005;352:2082–90.
35. Chang AB, Redding GJ, Everard ML. Chronic wet cough: protracted bronchitis, chronic suppurative lung disease and bronchiectasis. Pediatr Pulmonol 2008;43:519–31.
36. Donnelly D, Critchlow A, Everard ML. Outcomes in children treated for persistent bacterial bronchitis. Thorax 2007;62:80–4.

37. Freymuth F, Vabret A, Brouard J, et al. Detection of viral, Chlamydia pneumoniae and Mycoplasma pneumoniae infections in exacerbations of asthma in children. J Clin Virol 1999;13:131–9.

38. Esposito S, Blasi F, Arosio C, et al. Importance of acute Mycoplasma pneumoniae and Chlamydia pneumoniae infections in children with wheezing. Eur Respir J 2000;16:1142–6.

39. Thumerelle C, Deschildre A, Bouquillon C, et al. Role of viruses and atypical bacteria in exacerbations of asthma in hospitalized children: a prospective study in the Nord-Pas de Calais region (France). Pediatr Pulmonol 2003;35: 75–82.

40. Biscardi S, Lorrot M, Marc E, et al. Mycoplasma pneumoniae and asthma in children. Clin Infect Dis 2004;38:1341–6.

41. Varshney AK, Chaudhry R, Saharan S, et al. Association of Mycoplasma pneumoniae and asthma among Indian children. FEMS Immunol Med Microbiol 2009;56: 25–31.

42. Teig N, Anders A, Schmidt C, et al. Chlamydophila pneumoniae and Mycoplasma pneumoniae in respiratory specimens of children with chronic lung diseases. Thorax 2005;60:962–6.

43. Kjaer BB, Jensen JS, Nielsen KG, et al. Lung function and bronchial responsiveness after Mycoplasma pneumoniae infection in early childhood. Pediatr Pulmonol 2008;43:567–75.

44. Sutherland ER, Martin RJ. Asthma and atypical bacterial infection. Chest 2007; 132:1962–6.

45. Webley WC, Salva PS, Andrzejewski C, et al. The bronchial lavage of pediatric patients with asthma contains infectious Chlamydia. Am J Respir Crit Care Med 2005;171:1083–8.

46. Mills GD, Lindeman JA, Fawcett JP, et al. Chlamydia pneumoniae serological status is not associated with asthma in children or young adults. Int J Epidemiol 2000;29:280–4.

47. Korppi M, Paldanius M, Hyvarinen A, et al. Chlamydia pneumoniae and newly diagnosed asthma: a case-control study in 1 to 6-year-old children. Respirology 2004;9:255–9.

48. Webley WC, Tilahun Y, Lay K, et al. Occurrence of Chlamydia trachomatis and Chlamydia pneumoniae in paediatric respiratory infections. Eur Respir J 2009; 33:360–7.

49. Cunningham AF, Johnston SL, Julious SA, et al. Chronic Chlamydia pneumoniae infection and asthma exacerbations in children. Eur Respir J 1998;11:345–9.

50. Stallworth LE, Fick DM, Ownby DR, et al. Antibiotic use in children who have asthma: results of retrospective database analysis. J Manag Care Pharm 2005; 11:657–62.

51. Kozyrskyj AL, Dahl ME, Ungar WJ, et al. Antibiotic treatment of wheezing in children with asthma: what is the practice? Pediatrics 2006;117:e1104–10.

52. Johnston SL. Macrolide antibiotics and asthma treatment. J Allergy Clin Immunol 2006;117:1233–6.

53. Johnston SL, Blasi F, Black PN, et al. The effect of telithromycin in acute exacerbations of asthma. N Engl J Med 2006;354:1589–600.

54. Richeldi L, Ferrara G, Fabbri LM, et al. Macrolides for chronic asthma. Cochrane Database Syst Rev 2005;19(4):CD002997.

55. Strunk RC, Bacharier LB, Phillips BR, et al. Azithromycin or montelukast as inhaled corticosteroid-sparing agents in moderate-to-severe childhood asthma study. J Allergy Clin Immunol 2008;122:1138–44.

56. Esposito S, Bosis S, Faelli N, et al. Role of atypical bacteria and azithromycin therapy for children with recurrent respiratory tract infections. Pediatr Infect Dis J 2005;24:438–44.
57. Turnbaugh PJ, Ley RE, Hamady M, et al. The human microbiome project. Nature 2007;449:804–10.
58. Hilty M, Burke C, Pedro H, et al. Disordered microbial communities in asthmatic airways. PLoS One 2010;5:e8578.

Effects of Atypical Infections with Mycoplasma and Chlamydia on Asthma

Gregory Metz, MD[a], Monica Kraft, MD[b],*

KEYWORDS

- Atypical bacteria • Asthma • *Mycoplasma pneumoniae*
- *Chlamydophila pneumoniae* • Exacerbation • Antibiotics

Asthma is a common condition characterized by inflammation, intermittent airflow obstruction, and bronchial reactivity. There are many factors that contribute to the pathogenesis of asthma and play a role in exacerbations and disease severity. Examples include underlying host susceptibility, atopy, environmental exposures, and respiratory infections. Viruses such as rhinovirus, coronavirus, respiratory syncytial virus, and human metapneumovirus are frequently detected in patients with asthma flares and are believed to be the most common trigger for exacerbations.[1,2] However, there is emerging evidence to suggest that atypical bacterial infections are positively correlated with asthma exacerbations, chronic asthma, and severity of disease. This article discusses *Mycoplasma pneumoniae* and *Chlamydophila pneumoniae*, and reviews studies evaluating their possible role in asthma. Significant limitations due to difficulties with sampling and detection exist in evaluating atypical bacterial infections in the lung.

MYCOPLASMA PNEUMONIAE AND RESPIRATORY DISEASE

Mycoplasma pneumoniae is an atypical bacterium that is transmitted by contact with respiratory droplets. The average incubation period is 21 days. *M pneumoniae* is a frequent cause of respiratory disease in humans. The pathogenic mechanism of the bacterium involves its association or cytoadherence with the respiratory mucosa. The bacteria interact with the host cells through an attachment structure that is

Funding support?

[a] Department of Medicine, Division of Pulmonary, Allergy and Critical Care Medicine, Duke University Medical Center, 4309 Medical Park Drive, Durham, NC 27704, USA

[b] Department of Medicine, Division of Pulmonary, Allergy and Critical Care Medicine, Duke University Medical Center, Research Drive, MSRB M275, Durham, NC 27710, USA

* Corresponding author.

E-mail address: monica.kraft@duke.edu

composed of multiple subunits that bind to various host cell receptors including sulfated glycolipids.[3] Once attached, *M pneumoniae* induces the generation of superoxide radicals and inhibits catalase, leading to oxidative stress in the host cell. *M pneumoniae* infection also induces the production of proinflammatory cytokines such as tumor necrosis factor (TNF)-α and interleukin (IL)-8, in part through engagement of Toll-like receptors (TLRs).[3] Infection ultimately leads to various pathologic changes to the respiratory epithelium including loss of cilia, metabolic derangements, and sloughing.

The immune response to *M pneumoniae* is multifactorial and includes innate signaling through TLRs, opsonization, phagocytosis, and adaptive immune responses such as antibody production and activation of TH_{17} cells.[3] Clinically, some individuals clear the bacteria whereas others only partially eradicate it, leading to a chronic low-level infection. Evidence suggests that established allergic airway inflammation may hinder clearance of the pathogen. Using a mouse model, Wu and colleagues[4] found that TLR2 expression was down-regulated in the presence of allergic inflammation and *M pneumoniae* infection. Recently, Wu and colleagues[5] also reported that low-dose *M pneumoniae* infection enhanced underlying allergic lung inflammation and augmented the T-helper 2 (Th2) response to allergen. By contrast, high-dose *M pneumoniae* infection attenuated the allergic response. Furthermore, Hoek and colleagues[6] demonstrated that rodent mast cells release IL-4 when cocultured with *M pneumoniae*, suggesting that *M pneumoniae* infection may promote allergic inflammation. Lastly, Chu and colleagues[7] found that *M pneumoniae* infection of allergen-sensitized mice resulted in an increase in airway collagen deposition. These animal studies suggest that *M pneumoniae* infection in the lung may play a role in asthma development, pathology, and disease activity.

CHLAMYDOPHILA PNEUMONIAE AND RESPIRATORY DISEASE

Chlamydophila pneumoniae is an obligate intracellular pathogen that is transmitted by person-to-person contact through respiratory secretions. The incubation period is 3 to 4 weeks. Many individuals remain asymptomatic during *C pneumoniae* infection whereas others develop sinopulmonary disease. *C pneumoniae* exists in 2 forms, the replicating reticulate bodies and the infective elementary bodies. After being released into the extracellular environment, the elementary bodies interact with respiratory epithelial cells, leading to phagosome formation and subsequent intracellular replication. In the lungs, *C pneumoniae* infection has been shown to increase endothelial nuclear factor (NF)-κB with subsequent up-regulation of inflammatory adhesion molecules, chemokines such as IL-8, and platelet-derived growth factor.[8] Epithelial cell adhesion molecules are also increased, leading to an influx of inflammatory cells. In addition, *C pneumoniae* may participate in airway remodeling through promotion of fibroblast proliferation driven in part by IL-6 and other growth factors.[8] Similarly to *M pneumoniae* infection, the immune response to *C pneumoniae* is multifactorial and includes innate, humoral, and cell-mediated immune mechanisms.

Pulmonary infection with *C pneumoniae* may also contribute to asthma development and disease pathology. Chen and colleagues[9] infected BALB/c mice with *C pneumoniae* intranasally, and found that repeated infection increased IL-4 gene expression and airway subepithelial basement membrane thickening, both features of atopic asthma. Using a murine model, Blasi and colleagues[10] demonstrated that intranasal infection with *C pneumoniae* resulted in sustained airway hyperresponsiveness as measured by methacholine challenge with barometric plethysmography. Recently, Bulut and colleagues[11] established that *C pneumoniae* heat shock protein

60 (cHSP60) contributed to the development of acute lung inflammation in mice, and concluded that cHSP60 may play a role in both acute and chronic lung inflammation. These animal studies suggest a mechanism by which *C pneumoniae* infection in the lung may contribute to the development and pathologic manifestation of asthma.

DIAGNOSIS OF ATYPICAL BACTERIAL INFECTIONS

There are significant limitations and challenges in diagnosing atypical bacterial infections in the lung. Current techniques include culture, antigen detection, serology, and polymerase chain reaction (PCR). Culturing atypical bacteria is time-intensive and technically difficult. Other methods for detection include enzyme immunoassays (EIA), enzyme-linked immunosorbent assays (ELISAs), and microimmunofluorescence.[3] For *C pneumoniae*, detection of IgM antibodies typically at 2 to 3 weeks after infection or a fourfold increase in IgG antibodies in convalescent sera suggests acute infection. For *M pneumoniae*, the EIA is frequently used to compare acute and convalescent sera looking for a fourfold increase in antibody titers. PCR detection of atypical bacteria is more sensitive, but there is a lack of standardization and availability. In addition, the correlation between these different diagnostic tests is fairly low.[12] A definitive diagnosis may require invasive tissue sampling, which is infrequently performed. Due to the lack of standardized tests and discordance between detection methodologies, there are limitations in the ability to accurately detect atypical bacterial infections of the lung, which subsequently affects the conclusions that can be drawn from available studies evaluating the role of atypical bacteria and asthma. Emerging techniques such as multiplex PCR and microfluidic platforms for *M pneumoniae* may provide methods for fast and sensitive diagnosis.[13]

ATYPICAL BACTERIAL INFECTIONS AND ACUTE EXACERBATIONS

In many studies, atypical bacterial infections are positively correlated with acute asthma exacerbations. For years there have been reports of a potential link between atypical infections and asthma. In 1970, Berkovich and colleagues[14] examined children with asthma and found evidence of *M pneumoniae* infection in 18% of asthma exacerbations. In 2004, Johnston and Martin[15] reviewed 12 studies looking at *C pneumoniae* and *M pneumoniae* infections and acute asthma flares, and found that 9 of the 12 studies demonstrated an association between infection and exacerbations. Several studies supporting a role of atypical bacterial infections in asthma exacerbations are now discussed here.

In a study of 74 mild to moderate adult asthmatics with acute exacerbations, Allegra and colleagues[16] reported that 20% of subjects had seroconverted to one or more viral or atypical bacterial pathogens as evidenced by a fourfold increase in titers during the 6-month study period. Evidence of atypical bacterial infection was found in 11% of subjects, 88% of which were caused by *C pneumoniae.* In contrast, only 9% of subjects with acute exacerbations had evidence of viral infection. A limitation of the study was that PCR methodologies were not available for diagnosis.

Miyashita and colleagues[17] evaluated 168 adults with asthma exacerbations and 108 matched controls, and found a significant increase in *C pneumoniae* infection in the asthmatic group as well as an increase in *C pneumoniae*–specific IgG and IgA in the asthmatics as compared with controls. The investigators subsequently concluded that *C pneumoniae* infection may contribute to asthma exacerbations. Furthermore, Cunningham and colleagues[18] evaluated 108 children with asthma, and obtained nasal aspirates and sera if there was a significant decrease in peak flow or an increase in respiratory symptoms. Of note, children with recurrent exacerbations were more likely to remain PCR-positive for *C pneumoniae* and have more than 7 times greater levels of *C pneumoniae*–specific IgA levels. Cunningham and colleagues postulated that the higher antibody response to *C pneumoniae* in subjects with increased asthma flares compared with those with fewer exacerbations could represent an increase in prevalence of infection or differential immune response to the bacterium.

In 2002, Lieberman and colleagues[19] performed a prospective study looking at 100 patients who were admitted to the hospital for asthma exacerbations. Subjects younger than 18 years and those with evidence of infiltrate by chest imaging were excluded. Blood samples from the subjects and age-matched controls were obtained at admission and 3 to 5 weeks later for serologic testing. The frequency of acute infections with various pathogens including viruses, bacteria, and atypical bacteria were compared between the asthma and control groups. Significant findings include the detection of influenza A in 11% of asthmatics versus 2% of controls, and positive serologic tests for *M pneumoniae* in 18% of hospitalized asthmatics compared with 3% of controls. There was no difference in detection of *C pneumoniae* between the 2 groups. Again, the study is limited by serologic diagnosis of infections, but the investigators concluded that *M pneumoniae* infection is correlated with asthma exacerbations requiring hospitalization.

A prospective analysis of 58 patients presenting to the emergency department with an asthma exacerbation revealed serologic evidence of an acute atypical infection with either *C pneumoniae*, *M pneumoniae*, or both in 38% of subjects.[20] The investigators obtained peak flow measurements at presentation and spirometry at follow-up, and found a significant reduction in peak flow and forced expiratory flow in 1 second (FEV_1) in the asthmatic group with atypical bacterial infections compared with the asthmatics without atypical bacterial infection. In addition, those presenting with severe asthma as defined by an initial peak expiratory flow (PEF) of less than 50% of predicted were more likely to have serologic evidence of acute atypical bacterial infection, with an odds ratio (OR) of 4.29.[20] Specific limitations of the study that are addressed in the publication include difficulties with diagnosis using serology, small sample size, and use of percent predicted instead of personal best for peak flow recordings. Despite these limitations, the results support an association between atypical bacterial infections and increased functional impairment during acute asthma exacerbations.

To evaluate the role of atypical bacterial infections in pediatric asthma exacerbations, Biscardi and colleagues[21] prospectively studied subjects who were admitted to hospital with severe asthma flares. Nasopharyngeal samples were obtained at admission and evaluated for the presence of a variety of respiratory viruses and for *C pneumoniae* and *M pneumoniae*. Acute infection was diagnosed by either elevation of specific IgM at initial serology or a 4-fold increase in IgG titers at follow-up. The subjects were divided into 3 groups for data analysis. Group 1 included 119 subjects with acute exacerbation of asthma. Group 2 consisted of 51 subjects presenting with their first onset of wheezing. Group 3 comprised 152 controls with chronic, stable asthma without exacerbation in the previous 6 months and/or allergic rhinitis. In group 1, *M pneumoniae* was found in 24 subjects (20%) and *C pneumoniae* was detected in 4 (3.4%) subjects during exacerbation. In the new-onset wheeze group, *M pneumoniae* was detected in 26 subjects (50%), a statistically significant difference when compared with group 1, and *C pneumoniae* was identified in 4 (8.3%). In the control group, only 8 (5.2%) had evidence of *M pneumoniae*. At 1-year follow-up, 62% of subjects in group 2 who had been diagnosed with an atypical infection had recurrence of asthma compared with only 27% of noninfected subjects in that group. This study also supports the potential role of atypical bacterial infections during acute asthma exacerbations and, interestingly, demonstrated that *M pneumoniae* infection was present in a large proportion of children presenting with their first asthma attack.

One of the hallmarks of asthma exacerbations is increased mucous production. The asthmatic airway expresses increased levels of the major mucin protein MUC5AC compared with nonasthmatic controls. Kraft and colleagues[22] reported that airway epithelial cells from patients with asthma demonstrated increased MUC5AC expression following *M pneumoniae* infection. In their study, bronchoscopy with airway brushings was performed on 11 asthmatic subjects and 6 nonasthmatic controls with subsequent culture of airway epithelial cells at an air-liquid interface with and without *M pneumoniae*. MUC5AC mRNA and protein expression were measured using PCR and ELISA techniques. The investigators found a significant increase in MUC5AC mRNA and protein expression in the asthmatic cells that were exposed to *M pneumoniae* and that this increase was attenuated by coculture with an NF-κB or TLR2 inhibitor.[22] Kraft and colleagues subsequently postulated that the increased mucin expression in asthmatic epithelial cells in response to *M pneumoniae* likely involves TLR2 signaling and NF-κB activation. Similarly, Morinaga and colleagues[23] also found that *C pneumoniae* infection of airway epithelial cells led to an increase in MUC5AC expression that could be reduced by treatment with macrolides and ketolides. This study also concluded that both ERK (extracellular signal-related kinase) and NF-κB were involved in MUC5AC production triggered by *C pneumoniae*. Various human studies support the potential role of atypical bacterial infections in acute exacerbations of asthma.

ATYPICAL BACTERIAL INFECTIONS AND THE DEVELOPMENT OF ASTHMA

The data supporting the role of atypical bacterial infections in the development of asthma is less clear. Zaitsu[24] compared 103 first-time wheezing infants and toddlers with 64 healthy controls. Seroconversion to *C pneumoniae* was significantly higher in the wheezing subjects than in controls (44.7% and 17.2%, respectively). Among the wheezing patients, those who progressed to developing asthma were statistically more likely to have a family history of allergic diseases and higher total IgE. Furthermore, wheezing patients with *C pneumoniae* infection were also more likely to develop asthma than those without infection (relative risk 2.9).[24]

In 2000, Kim and colleagues[25] investigated whether *M pneumoniae* infection led to impaired lung function. Thirty-eight children hospitalized for *M pneumoniae* lung infection and 17 control children with *M pneumoniae* upper respiratory infections without lung involvement completed high-resolution chest computed tomography (CT) 1.0 to 2.2 years after infection. Of note, 37% of the *M pneumoniae* infection group compared with 12% of the control group exhibited abnormal CT findings including bronchial wall thickening and air trapping, which contributes to airflow obstruction.

A population-based adult cohort study followed subjects for 15 years and investigated whether *C pneumoniae* infection conferred a risk of developing asthma or reduced lung function as compared with those without serologic evidence of *C pneumoniae*.[26] Although atypical bacterial infection did not increase the risk for development of asthma, the investigators found that subjects with chronic *C pneumoniae* infection and nonatopic asthma experienced a faster decline in FEV_1 compared with other asthmatics without chronic infection. These findings suggest that atypical bacterial infections may contribute to the development of airflow obstruction. However, it must be noted that several published studies do not support an association between atypical bacterial infection and the development of new-onset obstructive lung disease.[27,28] Consequently, further studies are needed to clarify the role of atypical bacterial infections in the development of asthma.

ATYPICAL BACTERIAL INFECTIONS, CHRONIC ASTHMA, AND SEVERITY OF DISEASE

Several studies support a correlation between atypical bacterial infections and chronic stable asthma. In 2001, Martin and colleagues[29] looked for evidence of infection with either M pneumoniae or C pneumoniae by PCR in 55 patients with chronic asthma and nonasthmatic controls, and found that more than 50% of asthmatics were positive for atypical bacteria as compared with 9% of controls. PCR-positive asthmatics also had a greater number of tissue mast cells, which raises the possibility that atypical bacterial infection of a previously sensitized host might augment underlying allergic inflammation, a finding that Wu and colleagues[5] described in a murine model of allergic asthma. Gencay and colleagues[30] evaluated 33 adult subjects with chronic stable asthma and matched controls for serologic evidence of infection with C pneumoniae. Significant findings include evidence of chronic C pneumoniae infection, as defined by C pneumoniae–specific IgG of 1:512 or more and IgA of 1:40 or more, in 18.2% of asthmatics versus 3% of controls.

In addition, evidence suggests that atypical bacterial infections may also alter the severity of chronic asthma. In the review by Johnston and Martin[15] of atypical infections and asthma, 16 of 20 studies supported a role for atypical infections in chronic asthma and several found an association between infection and severity of disease. In 1998, Hahn and colleagues[31] described 3 steroid-dependent asthmatics with serologic evidence for recent C pneumoniae infection who were able to discontinue oral steroids following antibiotic therapy for atypical bacteria.

Although based on a small group, the investigators[31] questioned whether these subjects' atypical bacterial infection contributed to steroid dependency and severity of disease. This idea was further evaluated by Black and colleagues[32] who examined 619 asthmatics for serologic evidence of C pneumoniae infection and collected clinical information including severity of symptoms, number and frequency of hospitalizations, and use of asthma medications. The investigators found a correlation between the use of high-dose inhaled steroids with increased C pneumoniae IgG and IgA titers. In addition, those with elevated C pneumoniae IgG had lower FEV_1 compared with percent predicted. Although it is unclear whether the use of high-dose inhaled steroids is a risk factor for developing atypical bacterial infections in the lung, these findings highlight the possibility that atypical infections may influence the severity of chronic asthma. Black and colleagues[32] propose that proinflammatory cytokines such as TNF-α and RANTES (Regulated upon Activation, Normal T-cell Expressed and Secreted) induced by the infection may contribute to disease severity.

In a prospective study of a Finnish cohort, subjects with nonatopic asthma with serologic evidence of C pneumoniae experienced a faster decline in FEV_1 than matched asthmatics without infection.[26] In addition, Ten Brinke and colleagues[33] followed 101 severe asthmatics in a cross-sectional study and determined that nonatopic asthmatics with serologic evidence of C pneumoniae infection had significantly greater estimated decline in postbronchodilator FEV_1/vital capacity. Put simply, C pneumoniae infection worsened the airflow obstruction, which may be explained in part by infection-related airway remodeling and inflammation.[33] Cook and colleagues[34] measured antibody titers to C pneumoniae in 123 acute asthmatics and 1518 nonasthmatic controls who were admitted to hospital.[34] Although antibody titers suggesting acute infection were not different between the groups, C pneumoniae antibody titers suggesting prior infection were found in 34.8% of those with chronic, severe asthma compared with 12.7% of controls with adjusted odds ratio of 3.99.

Chlamydial antigens such as HSP60 are responsible for activation of the host inflammatory cascade in response to infection. Immune responses directed against cHSP have been associated with the development of various inflammatory conditions including ocular and pelvic disease. Hahn and Peeling[35] tested for antibody responses to a cHSP60 fragment in adult asthmatics and 52 nonasthmatic controls who were exposed to C pneumoniae, and found that immunoreactivity to the cHSP60 fragment was associated with increased airflow limitation as defined by lower postbronchodila tor FEV_1. It is postulated that host immune responses to cHSP may contribute to airway pathology, thus worsening disease severity. Several human studies including those outlined here suggest an association between atypical bacterial infections and severity of asthma.

EFFECTS OF ANTIBIOTICS ON ATYPICAL BACTERIA IN ASTHMA

Although studies suggest a role for atypical bacterial infections in asthma exacerbations, chronic asthma, and severity of disease, the use of antibiotics such as macrolides directed against them is still under investigation and is not routinely practiced. The mechanism by which antibiotics such as macrolides affect asthma is not well understood and is likely to be multifactorial. If atypical bacterial infections contribute to asthma, one can imagine how antibiotic-mediated clearance of the bacteria may be beneficial. The effects of macrolides likely extend far beyond their antimicrobial properties. Numerous studies have characterized the anti-inflammatory effects of macrolides, which include reduction in bronchial epithelial cell production of endothelin-1 (ET-1), down-regulation of adhesion molecules altering local inflammation, inhibition of airway mucous production, and reduction of proinflammatory cytokines such as IL-8.[36–39] Some of the human trials that have sought to investigate the effects of antibiotic therapy for atypical infections in asthma are outlined in this section.

Asthmatics with a current exacerbation were enrolled in a double-blind, placebo-controlled, randomized trial (TELICAST) investigating the efficacy of telithromycin during acute asthma flares.[40] A total of 278 acute asthmatics were enrolled and treated with standard care plus 10 days of either telithromycin or placebo. Culture, serology, and PCR techniques were used to evaluate for M pneumoniae or C pneumoniae. The primary outcomes were symptom scores and morning PEFs. Sixty-one percent of subjects had evidence of atypical bacterial infection. Symptom scores improved significantly in the treatment group; however, there was no difference in morning peak flows. Spirometry was obtained at various time points including baseline, end of treatment, and at 6 weeks. At the end of treatment, the FEV_1 improved by 0.63 L in the telithromycin group compared with 0.34 L in the control group ($P = .001$); however, this difference was no longer seen at 6 weeks. On subgroup analysis, it appears that the improvement in FEV_1 at the end of treatment compared with controls was only significant in those with evidence of atypical infection. The TELICAST trial demonstrated temporary clinical improvement following use of antimicrobials during asthma exacerbations, but raised many questions including who would benefit from therapy, whether the benefits outweigh potential adverse events, and the mechanism of action of antimicrobials in this setting.

Horiguchi and colleagues[41] examined the effects of sparfloxacin on 26 asthmatics with serologic evidence of C pneumoniae. The subjects were seen in an outpatient clinic and randomized to sparfloxacin, a respiratory quinolone that covers atypical bacteria, or no treatment for a total of 21 days. Of note, the treatment subjects reported a decrease in symptoms, less rescue medication use, and improved morning peak flows. Although it suggests that antimicrobial therapy can improve asthma, this study is limited by the small sample size and bias that may be introduced from non-blinded treatment. Black and colleagues[42] performed a randomized, double-blind, placebo-controlled trial (CARM study) evaluating the use of roxithromycin in asthmatics with serologic evidence of C pneumoniae. The study included 232 subjects who participated in a 2-week run-in period, 6 weeks of treatment with either roxithromycin or placebo, and 24 weeks of follow-up. The primary end points included asthma symptom scores and the change in mean PEF. Following treatment there was no difference in symptom scores, but the roxithromycin group experienced a greater increase in mean evening PEF (15 L/min) compared with placebo (3 L/min), which was no longer seen at 3 months. This trial demonstrated a transient effect on evening PEF following antibiotic therapy.

In 2001, Kraft and colleagues[43] studied the effects of clarithromycin on 55 subjects with chronic asthma. The subjects completed methacholine challenges, spirometry, chest radiography, and upper and lower airway sampling, which included PCR analysis for M pneumoniae and C pneumoniae. The subjects were randomized to receive clarithromycin or placebo for 6 weeks with subsequent evaluation of lung function and measurement of inflammatory mediators. Significant findings include evidence of M pneumoniae and/or C pneumoniae in 56% of asthmatics. PCR-positive treatment subjects experienced an increase in FEV_1 (2.50 ± 0.16 to 2.69 ± 0.19 L; $P = .05$) that was not found in PCR-negative subjects in the treatment group or in controls. The investigators analyzed bronchoalveolar lavage samples for cytokine expression, and found a reduction in TNF-α, IL-5, and IL-12 mRNA in the PCR-positive asthmatics treated with clarithromycin and a reduction in TNF-α and IL-12 mRNA in treated subjects who were PCR-negative. There were no changes noted in inflammatory cytokines in the placebo group. Kraft and colleagues concluded that clarithromycin improved lung function in patients with evidence of atypical bacteria in addition to reducing pulmonary inflammatory cytokines in both PCR-positive and -negative subjects.

Studies also support a beneficial role of macrolides in asthmatics that is independent of infection with atypical bacteria. Simpson and colleagues.[44] treated severe, refractory asthmatics without known M pneumoniae or C pneumoniae colonization with clarithromycin or placebo for 8 weeks and found improved quality-of-life scores and reduced sputum IL-8 in the treated subjects. The investigators speculated that macrolides may provide effective adjunctive treatment, especially for those with severe asthma and presumed neutrophilic disease, primarily because of their anti-inflammatory properties. Although some studies suggest a possible therapeutic benefit from use of antimicrobials in asthma, it remains unclear as to who would benefit from therapy and whether any improvement in lung function or symptoms can be sustained. The most recent Cochrane review in 2005 to evaluate the effects of macrolides for chronic asthma cited insufficient evidence to currently recommend their use.[45] This topic clearly requires further investigation to better understand the role of antimicrobial therapy in asthma.

SUMMARY

Taken together, these studies suggest that C pneumoniae and M pneumoniae infections are frequently present in acute exacerbations and chronic asthma. In addition, there is mounting evidence to suggest that atypical bacterial infections may also affect the severity of disease, although a causal role for the development of asthma has not been proved. Significant limitations exist in diagnosing atypical bacterial infections in the lung because of difficulties with sampling and lack of standardized detection methodologies. Numerous animal and human studies have outlined mechanisms by which atypical bacterial infections may contribute to airway obstruction through promotion of allergic airway inflammation and airway remodeling. Additional trials are needed to clarify the role of antimicrobials for atypical bacteria in asthma. As our understanding of the role of atypical infections in asthma expands, antimicrobial and anti-inflammatory therapies targeted for specific asthma phenotypes may provide new therapeutic options.

ACKNOWLEDGMENTS

The authors thank Dr Druhan Howell for contributing to this article.

REFERENCES

1. Newcomb DC, Peebles RS Jr. Bugs and asthma: a different disease? Proc Am Thorac Soc 2009;6(3):266–71.
2. Krishnan V, Diette GB, Rand CS, et al. Mortality in patients hospitalized for asthma exacerbations in the United States. Am J Respir Crit Care Med 2006;174:633–8.
3. Waites KB, Balish MF, Atkinson TP. New insights into the pathogenesis and detection of *Mycoplasma pneumoniae* infections. Future Microbiol 2008;3(6):635–48.
4. Wu Q, Martin RJ, Lafasto S, et al. Toll-like receptor 2 down-regulation in established mouse allergic lungs contributes to decreased mycoplasma clearance. Am J Respir Crit Care Med 2008;177:720–9.
5. Wu Q, Martin RJ, LaFasto S, et al. A low dose of *Mycoplasma pneumoniae* infection enhances an established allergic inflammation in mice: the role of the prostaglandin E2 pathway. Clin Exp Allergy 2009;39(11):1754–63.
6. Hoek KL, Cassell GH, Duffy LB, et al. *Mycoplasma pneumoniae*-induced activation and cytokine production in rodent mast cells. J Allergy Clin Immunol 2002; 109(3):470–6.
7. Chu HW, Rino JG, Wexler RB, et al. *Mycoplasma pneumoniae* infection increases airway collagen deposition in a murine model of allergic airway inflammation. Am J Physiol Lung Cell Mol Physiol 2005;289(1):L125–33.
8. Blasi F, Tarsia P, Aliberti S. *Chlamydophila pneumoniae*. Clin Microbiol Infect 2009;15(1):29–35.
9. Chen CZ, Yang BC, Lin TM, et al. Chronic and repeated *Chlamydophila pneumoniae* lung infection can result in increasing IL-4 gene expression and thickness of airway subepithelial basement membrane in mice. J Formos Med Assoc 2009; 108(1):45–52.
10. Blasi F, Aliberti S, Allegra L, et al. *Chlamydophila pneumoniae* induces a sustained airway hyperresponsiveness and inflammation in mice. Respir Res 2007; 8:83.
11. Bulut Y, Shimada K, Wong MH, et al. Chlamydial heat shock protein 60 induces acute pulmonary inflammation in mice via the toll-like receptor 4- and MyD88-dependent pathway. Infect Immun 2009;77(7):2683–90.
12. Kumar S, Hammerschlag MR. Acute respiratory infection due to *Chlamydia pneumoniae*: current status of diagnostic methods. Clin Infect Dis 2007;44(4):568–76.
13. Wulff-Burchfield E, Schell WA, Eckhardt AE, et al. Microfluidic platform versus conventional real-time polymerase chain reaction for the detection of

Mycoplasma pneumoniae in respiratory specimens. Diagn Microbiol Infect Dis 2010;67(1):22–9.

14. Berkovich S, Millian SJ, Snyder RD. The association of viral and mycoplasma infections with recurrence of wheezing in the asthmatic child. Ann Allergy 1970;28(2):43–9.

15. Johnston SL, Martin RJ. *Chlamydophila pneumoniae* and *Mycoplasma pneumoniae*: a role in asthma pathogenesis? Am J Respir Crit Care Med 2005;172(9): 1078–89.

16. Allegra L, Blasi F, Centanni S, et al. Acute exacerbations of asthma in adults: role of *Chlamydia pneumoniae* infection. Eur Respir J 1994;7(12):2165–8.

17. Miyashita N, Kubota Y, Nakajima M, et al. *Chlamydia pneumoniae* and exacerbations of asthma in adults. Ann Allergy Asthma Immunol 1998;80(5):405–9.

18. Cunningham AF, Johnston SL, Julious SA, et al. Chronic *Chlamydia pneumoniae* infection and asthma exacerbations in children. Eur Respir J 1998;11(2):345–9.

19. Lieberman D, Lieberman D, Printz S, et al. Atypical pathogen infection in adults with acute exacerbation of bronchial asthma. Am J Respir Crit Care Med 2003; 167(3):406–10.

20. Cosentini R, Tarsia P, Canetta C, et al. Severe asthma exacerbation: role of acute *Chlamydophila pneumoniae* and *Mycoplasma pneumoniae* infection. Respir Res 2008;9:48.

21. Biscardi S, Lorrot M, Marc E, et al. *Mycoplasma pneumoniae* and asthma in children. Clin Infect Dis 2004;38(10):1341–6.

22. Kraft M, Adler KB, Ingram JL, et al. *Mycoplasma pneumoniae* induces airway epithelial cell expression of MUC5AC in asthma. Eur Respir J 2008;31(1):43–6.

23. Morinaga Y, Yanagihara K, Miyashita N, et al. Azithromycin, clarithromycin and telithromycin inhibit MUC5AC induction by *Chlamydophila pneumoniae* in airway epithelial cells. Pulm Pharmacol Ther 2009;22(6):580–6.

24. Zaitsu M. The development of asthma in wheezing infants with *Chlamydia pneumoniae* infection. J Asthma 2007;44(7):565–8.

25. Kim CK, Chung CY, Kim JS, et al. Late abnormal findings on high-resolution computed tomography after *Mycoplasma pneumoniae*. Pediatrics 2000;105(2): 372–8.

26. Pasternack R, Huhtala H, Karjalainen J. *Chlamydophila (Chlamydia) pneumoniae* serology and asthma in adults: a longitudinal analysis. J Allergy Clin Immunol 2005;116(5):1123–8.

27. Korppi M, Paldanius M, Hyvarinen A, et al. *Chlamydia pneumoniae* and newly diagnosed asthma: a case-control study in 1 to 6-year-old children. Respirology 2004;9(2):255–9.

28. Larsen FO, Norn S, Mordhorst CH, et al. *Chlamydia pneumoniae* and possible relationship to asthma. Serum immunoglobulins and histamine release in patients and controls. APMIS 1998;106(10):928–34.

29. Martin RJ, Kraft M, Chu HW, et al. A link between chronic asthma and chronic infection. J Allergy Clin Immunol 2001;107(4):595–601.

30. Gencay M, Rüdiger JJ, Tamm M, et al. Increased frequency of *Chlamydia pneumoniae* antibodies in patients with asthma. Am J Respir Crit Care Med 2001; 163(5):1097–100.

31. Hahn DL, Bukstein D, Luskin A, et al. Evidence for *Chlamydia pneumoniae* infection in steroid-dependent asthma. Ann Allergy Asthma Immunol 1998;80(1):45–9.

32. Black PN, Scicchitano R, Jenkins CR, et al. Serological evidence of infection with *Chlamydia pneumoniae* is related to the severity of asthma. Eur Respir J 2000; 15(2):254–9.

33. Ten Brinke A, van Dissel JT, Sterk PJ, et al. Persistent airflow limitation in adult-onset non-atopic asthma is associated with serologic evidence of *Chlamydia pneumoniae* infection. J Allergy Clin Immunol 2001;107(3):449–54.
34. Cook PJ, Davies P, Tunnicliffe W, et al. *Chlamydia pneumoniae* and asthma. Thorax 1998;53(4):254–9.
35. Hahn DL, Peeling RW. Airflow limitation, asthma, and *Chlamydia pneumoniae*-specific heat shock protein 60. Ann Allergy Asthma Immunol 2008;101(6):614–8.
36. Takizawa H, Desaki M, Ohtoshi T, et al. Erythromycin and clarithromycin attenuate cytokine induced endothelin-1 expression in human bronchial epithelial cells. Eur Respir J 1998;12(1):57–63.
37. Kawasaki S, Takizawa H, Ohtoshi T, et al. Roxithromycin inhibits cytokine production by and neutrophil attachment to human bronchial epithelial cells in vitro. Antimicrob Agents Chemother 1998;42(6):1499–502.
38. Shimizu T, Shimizu S, Hattori R, et al. In vivo and in vitro effects of macrolide antibiotics on mucus secretion in airway epithelial cells. Am J Respir Crit Care Med 2003;168(5):581–7.
39. Takizawa H, Desaki M, Ohtoshi T, et al. Erythromycin modulates IL-8 expression in normal and inflamed human bronchial epithelial cells. Am J Respir Crit Care Med 1997;156(1):266–71.
40. Johnston SL, Blasi F, Black PN, et al. The effect of telithromycin in acute exacerbations of asthma. N Engl J Med 2006;354(15):1589–600.
41. Horiguchi T, Miyazaki J, Ohira D, et al. Usefulness of sparfloxacin against *Chlamydia pneumoniae* infection in patients with bronchial asthma. J Int Med Res 2005;33(6):668–76.
42. Black PN, Blasi F, Jenkins CR, et al. Trial of roxithromycin in subjects with asthma and serological evidence of infection with *Chlamydia pneumoniae*. Am J Respir Crit Care Med 2001;164(4):536–41.
43. Kraft M, Cassell GH, Pak J, et al. *Mycoplasma pneumoniae* and *Chlamydia pneumoniae* in asthma: effect of clarithromycin. Chest 2002;121(6):1782–8.
44. Simpson JL, Powell H, Boyle MJ, et al. Clarithromycin targets neutrophilic airway inflammation in refractory asthma. Am J Respir Crit Care Med 2008;177(2): 148–55.
45. Richeldi L, Ferrara G, Fabbri LM, et al. Macrolides for chronic asthma. Cochrane Database Syst Rev 2005;4:CD002997.

Index

Note: Page numbers of article titles are in **boldface** type.

Immunol Allergy Clin N Am 30 (2010) 587–592
doi:10.1016/S0889-8561(10)00094-9
0889-8561/10/$ – see front matter © 2010 Elsevier Inc. All rights reserved.

immunology.theclinics.com

United States Postal Service

Statement of Ownership, Management, and Circulation
(All Periodicals Publications Except Requestor Publications)

1. Publication Title	2. Publication Number	3. Filing Date
Immunology and Allergy Clinics of North America	0 0 6 – 3 6 1	9/15/10

4. Issue Frequency	5. Number of Issues Published Annually	6. Annual Subscription Price
Feb, May, Aug, Nov	4	$254.00

7. Complete Mailing Address of Known Office of Publication (Not printer) (Street, city, county, state, and ZIP+4®)

Elsevier Inc.
360 Park Avenue South
New York, NY 10010-1710

Contact Person
Stephen Bushing

Telephone (Include area code)
215-239-3688

8. Complete Mailing Address of Headquarters or General Business Office of Publisher (Not printer)

Elsevier Inc., 360 Park Avenue South, New York, NY 10010-1710

9. Full Names and Complete Mailing Addresses of Publisher, Editor, and Managing Editor (Do not leave blank)

Publisher (Name and complete mailing address)

Kim Murphy, Elsevier, Inc., 1600 John F. Kennedy Blvd. Suite 1800, Philadelphia, PA 19103-2899

Editor (Name and complete mailing address)

Patrick Manley, Elsevier, Inc., 1600 John F. Kennedy Blvd. Suite 1800, Philadelphia, PA 19103-2899

Managing Editor (Name and complete mailing address)

Catherine Bewick, Elsevier, Inc., 1600 John F. Kennedy Blvd. Suite 1800, Philadelphia, PA 19103-2899

10. Owner (Do not leave blank. If the publication is owned by a corporation, give the name and address of the corporation immediately followed by the names and addresses of all stockholders owning or holding 1 percent or more of the total amount of stock. If not owned by a corporation, give the names and addresses of the individual owners. If owned by a partnership or other unincorporated firm, give its name and address as well as those of each individual owner. If the publication is published by a nonprofit organization, give its name and address.)

Full Name	Complete Mailing Address
Wholly owned subsidiary of	4520 East-West Highway
Reed/Elsevier, US holdings	Bethesda, MD 20814

11. Known Bondholders, Mortgagees, and Other Security Holders Owning or Holding 1 Percent or More of Total Amount of Bonds, Mortgages, or Other Securities. If none, check box ☐ None

Full Name	Complete Mailing Address
N/A	

12. Tax Status (For completion by nonprofit organizations authorized to mail at nonprofit rates) (Check one)
The purpose, function, and nonprofit status of this organization and the exempt status for federal income tax purposes:
☐ Has Not Changed During Preceding 12 Months
☐ Has Changed During Preceding 12 Months (Publisher must submit explanation of change with this statement)

PS Form **3526**, September 2007 (Page 1 of 3 (Instructions Page 3)) PSN 7530-01-000-9931 PRIVACY NOTICE See our Privacy policy in www.usps.com

---

13. Publication Title	14. Issue Date for Circulation Data Below
Immunology and Allergy Clinics of North America	August 2010

15. Extent and Nature of Circulation			Average No. Copies Each Issue During Preceding 12 Months	No. Copies of Single Issue Published Nearest to Filing Date
a. Total Number of Copies (Net press run)			938	900
b. Paid Circulation (By Mail and Outside the Mail)	(1)	Mailed Outside-County Paid Subscriptions Stated on PS Form 3541. (Include paid distribution above nominal rate, advertiser's proof copies, and exchange copies)	446	406
	(2)	Mailed In-County Paid Subscriptions Stated on PS Form 3541 (Include paid distribution above nominal rate, advertiser's proof copies, and exchange copies)		
	(3)	Paid Distribution Outside the Mails Including Sales Through Dealers and Carriers, Street Vendors, Counter Sales, and Other Paid Distribution Outside USPS®	114	113
	(4)	Paid Distribution by Other Classes Mailed Through the USPS (e.g. First-Class Mail®)		
c. Total Paid Distribution (Sum of 15b (1), (2), (3), and (4))		▶	560	519
d. Free or Nominal Rate Distribution (By Mail and Outside the Mail)	(1)	Free or Nominal Rate Outside-County Copies included on PS Form 3541	75	55
	(2)	Free or Nominal Rate In-County Copies Included on PS Form 3541		
	(3)	Free or Nominal Rate Copies Mailed at Other Classes Through the USPS (e.g. First-Class Mail)		
	(4)	Free or Nominal Rate Distribution Outside the Mail (Carriers or other means)		
e. Total Free or Nominal Rate Distribution (Sum of 15d (1), (2), (3) and (4))		▶	75	55
f. Total Distribution (Sum of 15c and 15e)		▶	635	574
g. Copies not Distributed (See instructions to publishers #4 (page #3))		▶	303	326
h. Total (Sum of 15f and g)		▶	938	900
i. Percent Paid (15c divided by 15f times 100)			88.19%	90.42%

16. Publication of Statement of Ownership

If the publication is a general publication, publication of this statement is required. Will be printed
in the **November 2010** issue of this publication. ☐ Publication not required.

17. Signature and Title of Editor, Publisher, Business Manager, or Owner

Stephen R. Bushing

Stephen R. Bushing – Fulfillment/Inventory Specialist

Date
September 15, 2010

I certify that all information furnished on this form is true and complete. I understand that anyone who furnishes false or misleading information on this form or who omits material or information requested on the form may be subject to criminal sanctions (including fines and imprisonment) and/or civil sanctions (including civil penalties).

PS Form **3526**, September 2007 (Page 2 of 3)

Moving?

Make sure your subscription moves with you!

To notify us of your new address, find your **Clinics Account Number** (located on your mailing label above your name), and contact customer service at:

Email: journalscustomerservice-usa@elsevier.com

800-654-2452 (subscribers in the U.S. & Canada)
314-447-8871 (subscribers outside of the U.S. & Canada)

Fax number: 314-447-8029

Elsevier Health Sciences Division
Subscription Customer Service
3251 Riverport Lane
Maryland Heights, MO 63043

*To ensure uninterrupted delivery of your subscription, please notify us at least 4 weeks in advance of move.

Printed and bound by CPI Group (UK) Ltd, Croydon, CR0 4YY

03/10/2024

01040461-0013